CW01638045

'Switched On'

Embracing the Science of Nutrigenomic Medicine

Christine Houghton

PhD., BSc., R.Nutr.

Nutritional Biochemist

"Switched On" is dedicated to those seekers of truth who appreciate that good health is acquired and maintained by adopting the time-honoured principles of Nature.

Compact but rich in scientific evidence, this book's foundation is anchored in the principles of Nature but translated into the context of a 21st century lifestyle.

SPECIAL NOTE TO READERS
The information contained within this book is for education and information purposes. It is not intended to provide diagnosis or treatment of any medical condition, nor is it intended to replace the guidance and personalized treatment provided by a health professional. Any application of the information provided in this book is at the readers' discretion and sole responsibility.

Third Edition - Revised and Expanded | September, 2021.

National Library of Australia
Cataloguing-in-Publication data:

Houghton, Christine.
Switched On – Embracing the Science of Nutrigenomic Medicine

Bibliography.

Includes Table of Contents

ISBN: 978-0-6453009-0-1

TABLE OF CONTENTS

FOREWORD

Stepping Through the Looking Glass

For the longest time, I believed that the only thing I needed to know about Nutritional Genomics was how gene variants changed the way we respond to our environment. Knowing this, we could personalise what we eat, our lifestyle, our environment and our supplements to optimise pathways that may have been impacted by our genetic variability.

That was until I met Dr Christine Houghton and read the first edition of *Switched On*. Everything changed for me. I realised that I was missing half of the equation, that it was important to differentiate between nutrigenetics (*gene variants*) and nutrigenomics (*gene expression*). Although Nutrigenetics gives us insights into what we have inherited, Nutrigenomics teaches us how to use nutrition, nutraceuticals, and lifestyle to change gene expression, enabling the body to heal itself.

This was the answer I had been looking for - for two decades. I had always known that nutrition was incredibly powerful for healing - but I had never understood the science behind this power - or how to translate it into clinical practice. *Switched On* started me on this learning journey. It challenged everything I had learned about nutrition in my Dietetics degrees and it opened me up to a new world where small bioactive plant molecules could do great things.

Do not be fooled by the slimness of this book. Reading it will be like *Alice in Wonderland* stepping through the looking glass. It will change how you view nutrition forever; it will empower you as a practitioner to be better than ever before – or as a non-technical reader - or a patient, to take control of your own health, utilising the tools of Nature.

Dr Yael Joffe. PhD RD FACN
Co-Founder 3X4 Genetics

PREFACE

Ten years have elapsed since I wrote the first edition of *Switched On*. Although that decade has seen enormous advances in the development of Nutrigenomics and its practical application, the core principles as outlined in the first and second editions remain.

The third expanded edition retains those principles, although modified and condensed in parts to allow for three new chapters to be included without losing the conciseness of the book.

A significant part of my focus over the last 10 years has been on compiling and delivering educational programmes for clinicians. As co-author of *Advanced Translational Nutrigenomics* and *Foundations in Nutrigenomics,* I have been privileged to see clinicians across the globe applying these principles in their own clinics.

In my thirty years as a Clinician in Nutritional Medicine, I never lost sight of the power of food to beneficially modify human health. It's possible that my clinical approach to both disease prevention and treatment was reinforced early in my career because so few nutritional supplements existed in the 1970s. What we achieved clinically in that era had to be accomplished with food. Those principles still apply, although the supplement industry has done its best to convince its customers that our soil is so poor that *'there is nothing left in our food'.*

Whilst there is certainly some truth in the fact that excessive use of agricultural chemicals has added to the contaminant burden of food and has diminished its nutrient content, recent studies reaffirm the health benefits of a balanced diet rich in minimally-processed plant food.[1]

By contrast, there are so many condition-specific supplements available today that both clinicians and their patients may find it easier to swallow a few pills than to address the diet and lifestyle habits that are well-known to be major contributors to the development of disease.

Since leaving clinical practice and moving into research, I am more persuaded than ever that diet and lifestyle, the tools of Mother Nature, must form the foundation of all therapeutic or preventive programmes if we are to enjoy our very best possible health status based on our own unique genetic blueprints.

That brings me logically to the subject of Nutrigenomics and the roles played by specific food-derived molecules in favourably modifying the expression of health-promoting genes. In this vein, the science of the plant molecule, *sulforaphane* has featured heavily in my research endeavours over the decade since *Switched On* was launched; there is so much more that I have learned about this remarkable molecule.

The year 2019 saw the launch of *Gut Ecology & Metabolic Modulation* (G.E.M.M.), a clinical intervention protocol I developed to combine the principles you will read about briefly in *Chapter 13.* G.E.M.M. is a nutrition-based approach that incorporates the function of the gut microbiome along with the sciences of *Immunology, Cell Biology and Microbiology*. Complicated as that may sound, I describe G.E.M.M. by saying *"The science is complex but the implementation is simple."*

Even though this book is not about G.E.M.M. *per se*, I have included a few 'gems' that are easy to include in any personal nutrition routine. The role of the microbiome as a foundation for restoring health has become well-known in the last few years – so much so, that it makes me wonder why we didn't realise this much sooner!

I do hope you enjoy this *snapshot* of nutrigenomics, an evolving science that has completely changed the way we must address human health.

Christine Houghton PhD.,BSc.,R.Nutr.
Brisbane, Australia September, 2021.

INTRODUCTION

It's possible you are reading this book because you have a genuine interest in your health and ways of enhancing your wellbeing and preventing disease; so you know that your most valuable asset is good health. Many of us fail to appreciate this fact until we become sick. Today's society encourages us to spend much of our time in search of material wealth, yet this is clearly no substitute for good health.

Do you ever feel as though you have little or no control over your health? And that you get sick without ever knowing why? Perhaps you feel helpless in thinking that you are dependent on pharmaceutical medicines or even surgery to stay reasonably well? Do you seem to be ageing prematurely? If this is how you feel, you're not alone!

This book can help you to regain control of your health by showing you how to use the principles of *Nutrigenomics (pr. Nutri-gen-o-mix)*, a relatively new science which puts the spotlight of health care back on you as an individual and away from helpless dependency on modern medicine. This is not to say that we shouldn't take advantage of the countless marvels modern medicine has to offer. Many of the sophisticated diagnostic and life-saving techniques of modern medicine are nothing short of brilliant!

What's worth considering however, is that the ready availability of pharmaceutical medicines for virtually any symptom you can imagine has discouraged us from looking for our own answers in the way that our ancestors did. Every civilization has its own healing tradition and some of the plant foods and medicines used in these traditions have been the basis from which modern pharmaceuticals have been developed.

Many of these traditional medicines continue to be used today, not only in the countries of their origin but also globally by individuals looking for ways to improve their health or to prevent illness.

> *The real power of Nutrigenomics lies in the identification and application of powerful food-derived biomolecules capable of 'switching on' or 'turning up' certain genes associated with cellular health.*

For most of us, every cell of the human body has all the information it needs to remain healthy and this information is coded within the DNA of *every* gene in *every* cell. Once we learn how to 'tap into' this code and better understand how to send it the signals it needs, all sorts of distressing symptoms may disappear. This may be as simple as feeling less tired, experiencing fewer aches and pains, better digestion, a better mood - sometimes just a sense of 'feeling better'.

Although Nutrigenomics may also use plants as sources of medicine, it is not a branch of any traditional medicine we have ever known. Instead, Nutrigenomics is firmly anchored in modern science, yet is simple enough that we can all take advantage of its principles. Although it sits on a foundation of Nutrition Science, the real power of Nutrigenomics lies in the identification and application of powerful food-derived biomolecules capable of *'switching on'* and *'turning up'* certain genes associated with cellular health.

To learn how this extraordinary new science can give us so much more control over our health and wellbeing, *read on......*

CHAPTER ONE

Has modern medicine lost its way?

Tools seemingly needed to practice modern medicine have become highly sophisticated but also impossibly expensive. None of them however, has been sufficient to curb the accelerating growth in chronic disease. Populations globally continue to succumb to the '*Diseases of Civilization'*; cancer, heart disease, diabetes, osteoporosis and arthritic conditions, to name the most prevalent.

Medicine justifiably boasts its ability to transplant organs, reattach severed limbs and replace worn-out joints. Yet, the common ailments which afflict millions the world over continue to defy practitioners of modern medicine. Whilst pharmaceutical drugs provide relief from the symptoms of many of these day-to-day ailments, they do little, if anything, to arrest the cause. What's more, most of these medicines produce adverse effects sometimes more distressing to the individual than the symptoms of the original complaint.

Too often we look in the wrong places to find ways to be healthy – pharmaceutical drugs and surgery should be our very *last* option, not our first. Mankind has survived on this planet for millions of years, using only what Nature has provided – so, perhaps we don't need to make day-to-day health care so complicated, nor so impossibly expensive!

The practice of modern medicine as we know it today is associated with treatments based largely on the prescription of pharmaceutical drugs, some of which are vaccines. When such prescriptions fail, surgery is often the next level of treatment. Such treatments are not without risks.

Dr Barbara Starfield,[2] a professor in health policy and management at Johns Hopkins University in Baltimore Maryland, has published frightening statistics on deaths due to medical error in the United States. Her 2000 data show that each year there are around 12,000 deaths from unnecessary surgery, 7,000 deaths from medication errors in hospitals, 20,000 deaths from other errors in hospitals, 106,000 deaths from the adverse effects of medications prescribed in error and 80,000 deaths from hospital-acquired infection. This is a total of 225,000 deaths every year which are due to error or to adverse reactions to prescribed medication. More recent 2017 data[3] reveal that medical errors may account for as many as 251,000 deaths annually in the United States.

To put this into a different perspective, medical error, she says, constitutes the third leading cause of death in the U.S. after heart disease and cancer. These data are unlikely to be very much different in other developed countries. In Australia where I live, the data are quite similar on a per capita basis.

The leading causes of death 100 years ago were more likely to be the infectious diseases, tuberculosis and pneumonia. Improved hygiene and modern medicines have seen these deaths replaced by the chronic *degenerative and inflammatory* diseases. In the 2019 year, the combined effects of *heart disease, cancer* and *stroke* led to the death of 28 times more people than from influenza and pneumonia.(*Accessed 9.3.2021* https://www.cdc.gov/nchs/products/databriefs/db395.htm#section_4)

The degenerative diseases include the *wear and tear* diseases such as break down of the joints and clogging of the blood vessels with fatty plaque. The *inflammatory* diseases include arthritis (*pain, redness and swelling*) of the joints, asthma *(inflammation of the airways*) and cardiovascular disease (*inflammation of the blood vessels*).

Leading the Charge In more recent years, the term *Integrative Medicine* has been used to describe those conventionally-trained medical practitioners who integrate aspects of non-pharmaceutical medicine into their mainstream practices.

The U.S. National Institutes of Health (NIH) define Integrative Medicine as *"combining mainstream medical therapies and CAM [i] therapies, for which there is some high-quality scientific evidence of safety and effectiveness."* To the patient, it may appear as if the practitioner is trained as both a medical practitioner and a natural therapist, considered by many to be a distinct advantage.

Because Integrative Medicine stands outside the criteria for medical registration, an Integrative Medicine practitioner, although satisfying the necessary regulatory criteria to practise mainstream medicine, is not required to meet standards in Integrative Medicine. The internal standards which these practitioners have established to train and credential their members are not acknowledged by governing authorities; nor are they known or understood by consumers. As a result, a consumer has no way of knowing how knowledgeable or competent an Integrative Medicine practitioner may be.

Regardless of any such current barriers to practice, those forward-thinking Integrative Medicine clinicians who have stepped outside conventional practice to embrace evidence-based alternatives are in huge demand. I personally know many such clinicians to have *'waiting-list'* practices; surely this illustrates what consumers are really seeking.

Interestingly, medical practitioners in some universities must still take the '*Hippocratic Oath'* before they can practise medicine. Hippocrates was a doctor and teacher of medicine some 2,500 years ago and is referred to as the *'Father of modern medicine'*. He is credited with saying, "*Let food be thy medicine and medicine be thy food."*

Although Hippocrates' claim that *food and medicine are interchangeable* seems overly simplistic in the 21st century, there are elements of this philosophy which are still relevant today. This is especially so in the science of Nutrigenomics, as we will see later.

---

[i] CAM - *Complementary and Alternative Medicine*

CHAPTER TWO

Why do we get sick?

If you've only ever enjoyed good health, you may have never given a thought to the question, "Why do some people get sick and yet others remain healthy?" If you are like most of us, from time to time you will have some experience of sickness but as the years advance, you might notice that your health deteriorates inexplicably. You may become more breathless, you may develop recurrent indigestion, perhaps you feel stiff and sore when getting out of bed in the mornings or you may need frequent naps and so on.

All little things in themselves but nevertheless, they are indicators that things are changing on the inside in ways that limit your experience of life. And then to make things worse, a visit to the GP followed by various tests, shows that those little 'signs' are actually just the tip of the iceberg. The GP may tell you that you have all sorts of things going wrong. High blood pressure, high blood cholesterol and higher-than-normal blood glucose all point to a significant risk of your developing diabetes, heart disease or both! Next thing, you are prescribed pharmaceutical drugs to lower the blood pressure, the cholesterol and the glucose, along with a suggestion to eat a low-fat diet and walk more often. How did this suddenly happen, you wonder. "I eat well", you say "and I don't need to do any extra walking – I'm busy all day – I never have a minute to myself."

Mostly, we just accept that this is how things are – that this is the hand of cards we were dealt at birth. You might remember that your parents or grandparents suffered from some of these same conditions and that you should probably expect to have inherited the same tendencies to disease.

To reassure the patient (and perhaps their own ignorance?), it is not uncommon for GPs to 'justify' the presence of a patient's illness by stating that he or she inherited the disease from one or both parents – and yet this is patently untrue because GPs don't typically do genetic tests to determine if diseases run in families.

Although it is now possible to obtain such genetic tests, especially if you are prepared to arrange and pay for them yourself, such tests are still *largely*[ii] the domain of research scientists, not clinicians. It might seem a logical assumption but is laying blame on one's genetic heritage necessarily the correct – or only explanation?

> *Mostly, we just accept that this is simply how things are – that this is the genetic hand of cards we were dealt at birth.*

So, if the disease is not inherited, why does the same disease appear to run in families? We've all seen families where the same disease seems to afflict many of its members. Is the cause genetic – or do families adopt the same poor lifestyle habits from one generation to the next?

But let's stop talking about disease and consider how it may be possible for us to take back control of our own health.

[ii] A technique known as Gene Expression Profiling, still very much in its infancy, investigates a range of genes which act as markers of an individual's likely functional weaknesses. Once these weaknesses have been biochemically identified, the patient may be prescribed a programme to modify the way certain genes are being expressed. The recommendations are based primarily on providing tailored nutritional, exercise and other lifestyle solutions to redress the imbalances created by inefficiently-functioning genes. Gene Expression Profiling, as long as it also makes appropriate recommendations for change, can help put control for health and wellbeing back into the hands of the individual.

CHAPTER THREE

Looking inside our body's cells for answers

Sometimes the concepts we think are the most complicated are really very simple. *'Healthy cells lead to a healthy body'* is a simplified message which tells us that if we know how to take care of each of our 50 trillion cells, our health will look after itself! So, if we know how to look after *one* cell, we know how to care for them *all*. Probably overly-simplistic but nevertheless, true!

To better understand how we can use Nutrigenomic principles to benefit our own health, let's take a microscopic journey deep inside a typical human cell. Once we know how a cell works, we can more readily appreciate how things can go wrong – but more importantly what we can do to improve cellular function - so that things go right! What benefits one cell can benefit *all* our cells. When all our cells function at their peak, we have reached our highest state of good health. And that should be our goal; to achieve our individual highest possible state of cellular function. The key here is that *we don't necessarily need to name* diagnosed diseases – the principles are the same, regardless.

Now let's explore some of the marvels of a typical human cell. We'll start with the membrane which could be likened to the 'skin' of the cell.

Cell Membrane - the cell's 'skin' Each cell is surrounded by a protective membrane which preferentially lets in water, oxygen, food and other molecules. Certain molecules simply 'flow' into the cell, whilst others need to be pumped in, using energy the cell has harnessed from food molecules. In the same way, the cell's membrane has a range of complex mechanisms for pumping waste materials out.

Mitochondria - the cell's *'Power Station'* Inside the cell are tiny, specialised bodies called mitochondria *(pr. my-toe-kon-dree-a)* which are the 'power stations', producing the energy the cell needs to perform all its functions. If the mitochondria aren't functioning properly, our cells can't produce sufficient energy to behave normally. Without adequate energy, practically anything can go wrong – and often does!

When your cells are sluggish because of lack of energy production, you will probably feel sluggish too! Sometimes this sluggishness within the cell can be because waste materials aren't being removed efficiently; sometimes, it is because the cell isn't receiving the food molecules it needs. This is one of the areas in which we can exert control; the foods we choose to eat have a direct impact on how our cells produce energy. Certain foods will enable the cell to function at its best while over-processed and refined foods which have lost many of their nutrients will deprive the cell of what it needs, thereby leading to abnormal function. Unprocessed or minimally-processed whole foods are essential for optimal energy production.

Nucleus – the cell's database Just as important as the mitochondria is the cell's nucleus, a large protective sac which holds our genes. Our genes, which are made up of long paired strands of DNA, store our unique *database* of genetic information. This database could be likened to your own personalised *Instruction Manual* – except that it contains so much information that it is more like an entire library than a single book!

As well as housing the *database* of information about you, the nucleus is responsible for the cell's reproductive system. Cells are said to *replicate* by dividing into two new identical cells at defined intervals. This process is controlled by the DNA.

This is incredibly significant to our health and wellbeing because when healthy cells divide, two new healthy cells are produced. However, when the DNA has become damaged, the new cells will carry that defect onto the next generation of cells. This sets the scene for ongoing patterns of disease which can be difficult to reverse; in other words, *chronic disease* can be the result.

The DNA has remarkable ability to repair such damage – to a point – but a lifetime of accumulated damage can sometimes overwhelm the cell's natural repair processes. This is where powerful *nutrigenomic* compounds as well as nutrients like folate and Vitamin B12 found in certain foods can help the DNA to protect and repair itself.

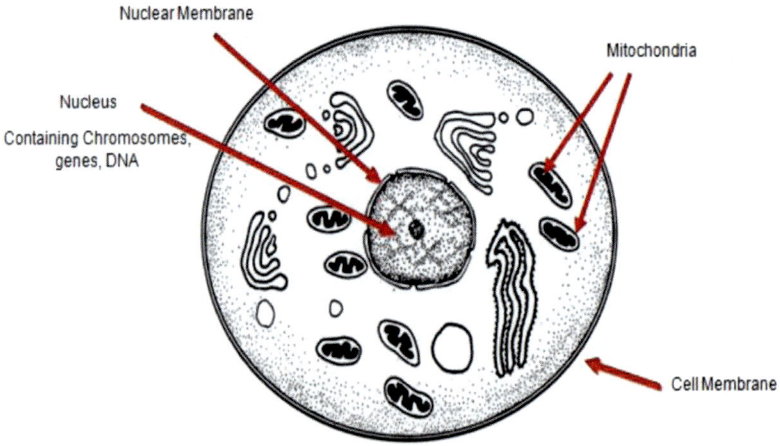

Figure 1: The Human Cell and its Organelles

The Cytoplasm The cytoplasm is a bit like the 'soup' in which the various cellular structures are suspended. However, this 'soup' is more than just part of the cell's structure; it is a rich source of thousands of essential chemical substances, all playing their own indispensable roles in maintaining normal cell function.

The chemical reactions occurring in the cytoplasm are enormously complex, with intricate signalling pathways providing instructions to the cell on a *moment-to-moment* basis. Each cell is a marvel in its own right – but just imagine how much more remarkable it is that the entire 50 trillion of our cells can function interactively for an entire lifetime!

CHAPTER 4

DNA, Genes and Chromosomes

Now before we explore the really exciting concepts that you can directly relate to your own health, let's zoom into the nucleus and take a closer look at the structures there. Sometimes, the terms *DNA, genes* and *chromosomes* are used interchangeably but they are in fact quite distinct entities. As a scientist, I find the intricacies of human cells fascinating. If you're not familiar with these concepts, I hope you enjoy this brief glimpse.

The DNA The cell's *database* which contains the code for absolutely everything about you starts with just four molecules, called *base pairs*, abbreviated as A, T, C and G. These base pairs are arranged like the steps in a spiral staircase with the hand-railing coiled in long strands.

This cabled structure is known as DNA and has been described as *'the double helix'* because of its characteristic helical shape.

Each person's DNA is unique to that individual. One strand of DNA is inherited from the mother and the other from the father. These are the complex molecules which determine everything we inherit – the colour of our eyes, our adult height, whether we can run fast, all our strengths and weaknesses.

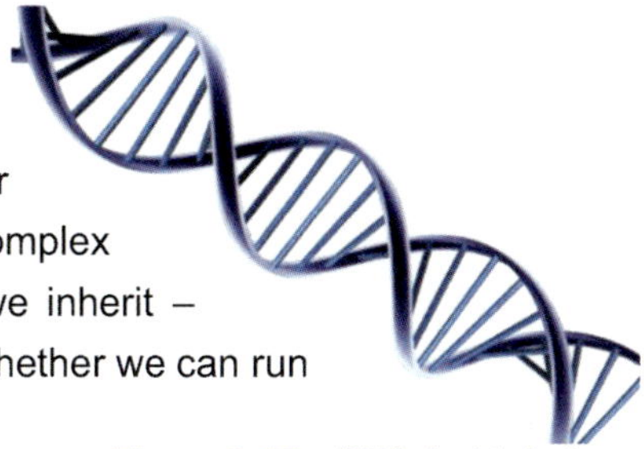

Figure 2: The DNA double helix joined by specific base pairs.

In fact, everything we inherit is coded here.

Of course, some of these factors such as eye colour and facial bone structure can't be changed because these genes are permanently *'switched off'* after birth. But of course, these genes can be inherited by the offspring, confirming what we readily observe when we see children who look like their parents.

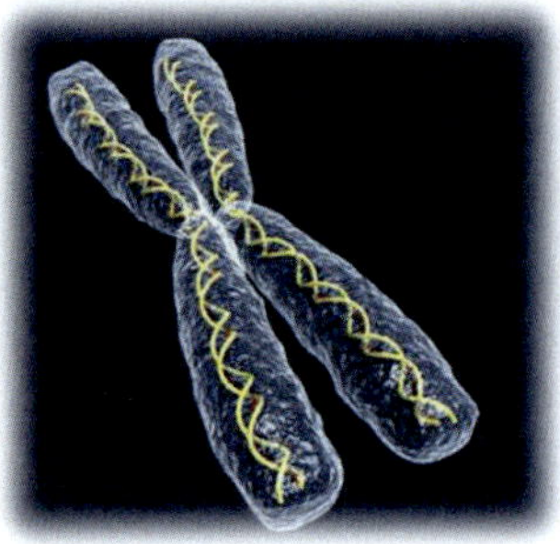

Figure 3: A single chromosome with the DNA double helix visible.

Scientists are now learning that we *do have control* over many of our very important genes and the way they can be expressed[iii]. Learning how to send the *right* messages to our genes is an important theme of this book. Equally important is the need to ensure that we don't send the *wrong* messages to our genes.

The Chromosomes The 25,000 or so human genes are contained in 23 pairs of non-identical chromosomes. The coiled DNA double helix is clearly seen within the chromosome in the illustration in Figure 3.

The Genes Even though the double helix is a continuous structure within each chromosome, at various intervals, a section of the DNA code contains a 'stop sign', signalling the end of the section of code for one gene - and the start of the code for another. Each of these separate sections is a single gene and each contains the code to tell the cell to make just one specific protein. So, when the gene is *'switched on'*, the code can be read and the cell makes a quantity of that particular protein.

[iii] When a gene is *'expressed',* this describes what happens when a gene is *'switched on'. 'Switching on'* or *'turning up'* a gene activates mechanisms which enable a specific protein to be produced. The gene contains the exact code for that protein – a bit like a recipe to tell the cell's 'machinery' the ingredients and the method to make it correctly.

And when the cell registers that it has made enough of the protein, the gene is then switched to the *'off'* position. Very clever, don't you think?

How these genetic 'switches' regulate insulin The glucose-regulating substance *insulin* is a good example of how this works. After a meal, when we have increasing amounts of glucose in the bloodstream, the cells of the pancreas detect this increase and switch the *insulin* gene to the *'ON'* position. When the right level of glucose is reached, the *insulin* gene is switched off. This is what we mean when we say that the cell is *intricately regulated,* switching genes on and off as the cell requires. No medicine can exert any such impressive regulatory control on cells.

The diagram in Figure 4 below shows the chromosomes containing long strands of DNA, which themselves show the genes that make up the chromosome. A gene which has been irreversibly damaged is said to contain a *mutation.* Mutations are often the fore-runner to the development of serious diseases such as cancer. However, not all mutations are harmful and are often Nature's way of allowing us to adapt over generations to changes in our environment.

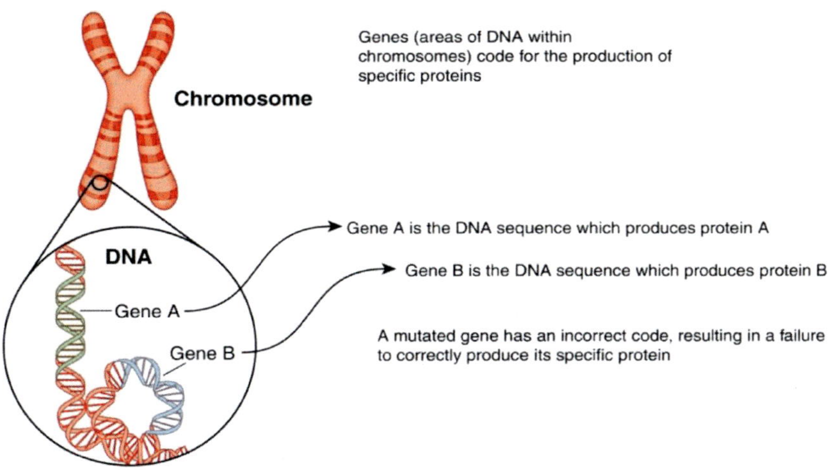

Figure 4: Each double-stranded DNA molecule is made up of individual genes. The genes contain the code for making a protein. Each of our 23 pairs of chromosomes contains tightly-wound chains of DNA which must be partially unwound for the code to be read.

CHAPTER 5

Nutrigenomics

– a new paradigm in health care

Scientists who completed the mapping of the human genome in around 2003[iv] identified around 25,000 genes which contain the individual genetic code for each of us. This number turned out to be surprisingly few genes, given the apparent sophistication of humans compared to many simpler animal species which have many more genes than humans.

In the following year, 2004, the term *Nutrigenomics* was coined, as the science that explains how foods (nutrients) interact with our genes (genomics). You can think of *Nutrigenomics* as *'your food talking to your genes'*. Whilst good food and lifestyle choices send 'healthy' messages to our genes, poor choices can damage the DNA in our genes, *'jamming up'* the cell's functions and clogging them with toxic by-products. If this process is ongoing day after day, disease will be the inevitable consequence.

It then became apparent that there was another layer of complexity, the *Epigenome*, which provided a form of modifiable chemical code within the cell's genetic material. *Epigenetics* is a 'sister' discipline to *Nutrigenomics* and later we will explore some of the fascinating aspects of this emerging discipline. Following the completion of the Human Genome Project, research into these relatively new scientific disciplines has become extremely relevant to human health. *Epigenetic* changes to the DNA are a bit like adding detachable paper clips here and there, making subtle but heritable changes to gene expression.

[iv] Known as the Human Genome Project

From the very first contact a new baby has with its mother's milk or colostrum[v], signals are being sent to the baby's genome. There can be lifetime consequences to infants (and *their* offspring) who are fed over-processed foods early in life; changes to the child's *epi*genome acquired during its lifetime can be passed down to subsequent generations.

Each of us in our pre-reproductive years has a huge responsibility to take care of the genome our future children and grandchildren will inherit. Rather sobering, isn't it, especially when our youthful pre-reproductive years are often spent abusing our bodies in ways that are pushing our cells to their absolute limits?

The burgeoning science of Nutrigenomics in many ways helps us to understand how human health has evolved over millions of years, slowly and constantly adapting to changes in our environment. As environmental factors changed over long periods of time, human cells gradually adapted. Such natural adaptation literally takes 'thousands and even millions of years' to occur.

Many scientists contend that, because of modern technology, Mankind has been exposed to such extraordinary change even in the last few hundred years that it has not been possible for us to adapt fast enough. Perhaps we have come to the 21st century dressed in Stone Age bodies!

The human genome knew nothing of the refined sugars which have become an integral part of modern dietary intake in most countries. Sugar intake in the American diet has increased by about 50% since the 1970s, largely due to massive increases in the use of high-fructose corn syrup (HFCS) in aerated beverages.[4]

Figure 5 shows the massive increase in sugar intake over the last 200 years, a period which is equal to about eight generations of ready access to refined sugar. This has simply not been long enough for our cells to

---

[v] **Colostrum** is the early mammary gland secretion. Most species will generate colostrum within one day of giving birth. Colostrum is rich in antibodies which provide immediate immune protection to the newborn.

have adapted. The pattern shown here does not reflect such changes in the United States alone; the pattern is now common across the globe.

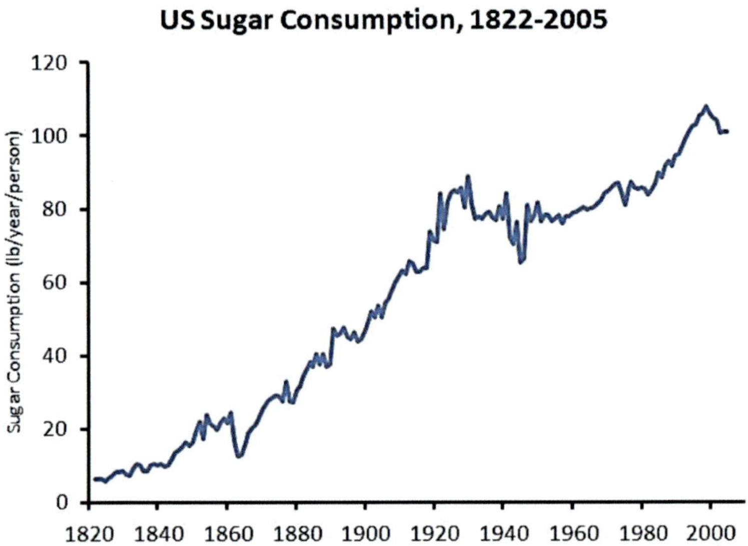

Figure 5: Data compiled by Dr Stephan Guyenet http://www.stephanguyenet.com/

In addition, the bewildering array of modern chemical additives now found in our food supply is unfamiliar to our cells. The cells can become easily overburdened by trying to detoxify the many thousands of foreign chemicals to which our genome is now exposed. Failure to detoxify will result in serious or fatal damage to the cell's delicate mechanisms.

One of the valuable lessons we have learned from Nutrigenomic Science is that if we were to eat a *plant-rich mixed diet* to which humans are well-adapted, our detoxification processes would function as they should. As an extension to this principle, Nutrigenomic Science has also helped us to identify which plant molecules have the greatest ability to activate the genes that code for the detoxification processes. It is these detoxification enzymes that allow us to effectively break down unwanted chemical residues, therefore preventing them from harming our cells.

One of the most extraordinary of these nutrigenomic molecules found in food is Sulforaphane *(pr. Sul-4-a-Fane).* Sulforaphane has such remarkable properties that we have devoted a large part of this book to its role in human health. Sulforaphane and other *nutrigenomic* compounds activate the *'switches'* within the cytoplasm of the cell. These *switches*, as we will see later, are then able to *'switch on'* or *'turn up* 'lazy' genes and *'switch off'* or *'turn down'* the overactive genes. As a result of the influence of such nutrigenomic compounds, cells which have lost their ability to properly regulate important functions can again work more efficiently, if not perfectly.

Detoxification of unwanted chemical substances is an essential function of all cells.[5] In fact, optimal detoxification is one of the most important ways in which cells can protect themselves against developing cancer. Sulforaphane has been shown to have remarkable potential in this role.[6]

Nutrigenomics has opened up a whole new understanding of the role of food in health. Where we once thought that food was just a source of building blocks like proteins, fats and carbohydrates plus essential vitamins and minerals, we now know that food is much more. It provides a huge 'library' of information which is continuously *'talking to our genes'*. It has been estimated that foods contain around five to ten thousand different substances.[7] Every one of these which can be absorbed into our cells has the potential to interact with the function of our cells.

Nutrigenomics has shown us that certain food molecules have very powerful effects, activating the cellular 'switches' that can significantly influence the internal health of the cells and their ability to defend and repair themselves.

Equally, we know that there are other foods such as the fats found in foods fried at high temperature that send different types of signals to our cells. Signals from such foods can *turn up* the genes which promote inflammation and destruction within the cells. Similarly, potentially-toxic chemical food additives and agricultural residues found in our food supply are continuously sending *'unfriendly'* messages to our DNA.

There is nothing new about the fact that some foods are *'good for us'* and other foods are *'bad for us'*. What's new is that a *handful* of particular food molecules has been identified as having exceptional cell-protective properties. When we incorporate these into our daily routine, we can maximise the benefit these remarkable substances can have on our own cells. And if every single one of your cells is healthy, *YOU* will be healthy!

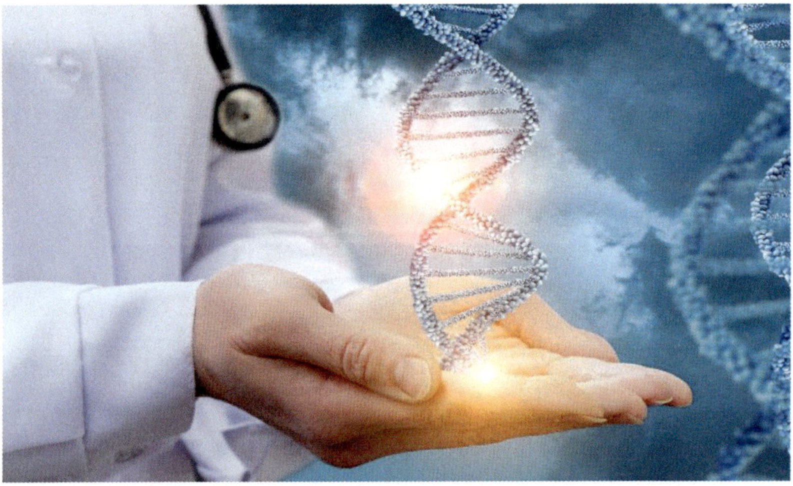

Figure 6: Your ability to take care of your cellular DNA is virtually in the palm of your hand!

Nutrigenomics has given us a much clearer understanding of how we can control the way our own cells work. By selecting the most powerful of the food molecules to be regular *'visitors'* to our cells, we can take over a significant level of control of the way our cells function.

Food then becomes so much more than a way of satisfying the palate or the appetite, pleasant as that might be. Nor is food just a way of obtaining calories or even vitamins or minerals.

Food is a *signalling system*, so that every choice we make sends a message to our cells. Do we choose to send the signals that are destructive to the cell – or those which optimise the cell's function?

Can you see that we are on the cusp of a whole new paradigm in health care – one in which you, as the sole owner of *YOUR* body can take back control of your health? This gives you the choice to be well – or to be plagued by illness. To a much larger extent than you may have imagined, we humans have significant control over our own health.

Pharmaceutical drugs are often the first approach to dealing with a health issue or even a diagnosed disease. Just as foods send signals to our cells, so too do pharmaceutical drugs. Using drugs as a first approach can be much like using a sledge-hammer to insert a thumb tack; it results in all sorts of collateral damage. Pharmaceutical medicines are simply not specific enough to make a correction in the cell's function without producing an array of undesirable other effects we call *side effects.* The side effects occur because the drug is just not sophisticated enough to single out the one effect it is designed to produce.

Compare this to being able to select a *nutrigenomic* compound capable of *'switching on'* hundreds of cell-protective genes at the same time; this is surely an opportunity to acknowledge the marvels of Nature! Such nutrigenomic substances are like the conductors of an orchestra, sending continuous subtle signals to the musicians so that the finished performance is perfectly-synchronised. Such is the magnificent and complex function of human cells; we are just beginning to comprehend their intricacies.

So, why would you choose a sledge-hammer when Nature's approach is so magnificently coordinated, gentler and precisely targeted?

By understanding the real power of *nutrigenomically-active* substances superimposed on the foundation of a healthy lifestyle, you can literally take back control of your own health. You no longer need to feel a helpless dependence on the sometimes sophisticated (but often clumsy) tools of modern medicine - the pharmaceutical drugs and surgery!

Is there a way that I can learn about my own DNA code? At around the time that the mapping of the human genome was completed, gene testing laboratories began offering individuals the opportunity to obtain a report with limited information about their DNA code. The early reports were of limited use but as the years have gone by, these reports have become very much more sophisticated. Some companies offer these reports directly to the consumer but to be clinically useful, most of the information really needs to be interpreted by a clinician who has been trained in both Nutrigenetics (*the study of how gene abnormalities affect the way food is metabolised)* and Nutrigenomics (*the study that identifies food molecules that can influence the expression of individual genes).*

Identifying Variations in our Genes Our DNA exists in long chains with two complementary chains intertwined. These chains are made up of combinations and patterns of just four nucleotide bases; they are shown in Figure 7 below abbreviated to the four letters, C, G, T and A. It's a bit like having an alphabet with only four letters – but with the letters arranged in groups of three. For our purposes here, these technicalities don't really matter.

We often refer to *gene variants* and this is like having a spelling mistake somewhere in the chain. The image below shows what happens when three different people have a different 'spelling mistake' at the same point in the DNA chain. These single 'spelling mistakes' are called *Single Nucleotide Polymorphisms*, abbreviated as SNPs – and pronounced

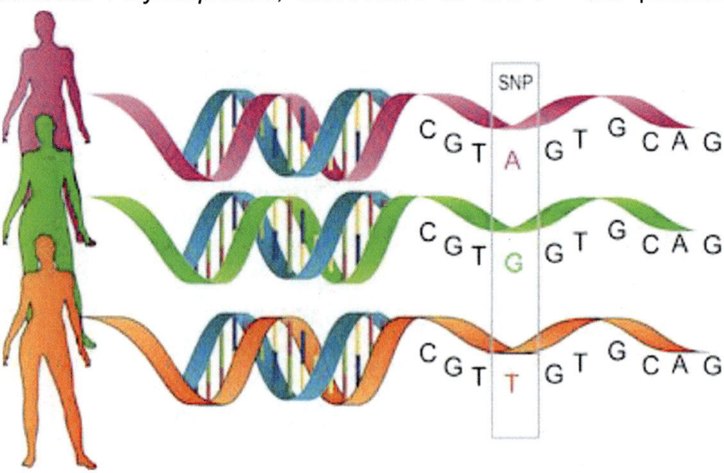

Figure 7: A single nucleotide base in the DNA chains making up a gene is like a 'spelling mistake'.

'SNIPS'. Each of us is thought to have been born with about four to five million SNPs, creating an enormous number of subtle differences across human populations, even in the same family.

Just like a spelling mistake we may make in writing a word, the word is still recognisable – but the gene may behave slightly differently from the version we consider to be the 'normal variant'. These SNPs don't stop the gene from working – they just make certain processes more or less efficient.

SNPs have very subtle effects on the way our body chemistry functions. For example, such subtle changes in our genes may determine whether our cells can detoxify waste materials efficiently when compared to the normal variant. SNPs in the genes that code for your antioxidant enzymes may modify your ability to neutralise (*or quench*) the free radical species that can lead to cell damage.

Knowing the SNPs that affect the core functions of your cells is very useful information. For example, if you knew that you carried a SNP in the gene that codes for the primary antioxidant enzyme, *Superoxide dismutase,* you could modify your diet and lifestyle to accommodate this. We could think of these SNPs as being *lazy* genes. Some which we term *homozygous* SNPs are extremely lazy and others we term *heterozygous* are moderately *lazy.*[vi]

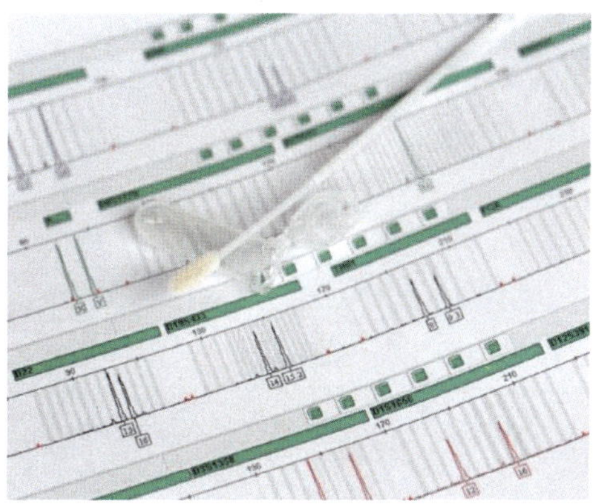

[vi] If the *spelling mistake* occurs in both strands of the DNA, we say the person carries a *homozygous* SNP in that gene (homo = both the same). If there is only one *spelling mistake*, we use the term *heterozygous polymorphism (or SNP)*

How is this information useful? Each of us is born with our own array of *SNPs* and it might be easy to think we are stuck with whatever weaknesses these SNPs confer on cell function. [8] But this is where Nutrigenomics comes in - and it is a very good news story! The science of Nutrigenomics has identified certain food molecules and lifestyle habits that can increase the activity of the 'lazy' genes.

When you have a genetic report that shows you which genes certain SNPs, a Nutrigenomics specialist clinician would immediately see where your system is likely to have its major weaknesses. His or her job then is to advise you on specific foods that are known to enhance the function of the *'lazy'* genes. Scientists say the food molecule *upregulates* the gene.

What tissue sample does a Nutrigenetic Test use? To find out what SNPs you carry in your own genome, you would send a sample of your DNA to a genetics lab. Such labs will provide you with a kit that contains a tiny circular brush that you use to brush around the inside of your cheek tissue. In so doing, some of the cells come off on the brush and then the brush is sealed in the secure tube supplied.

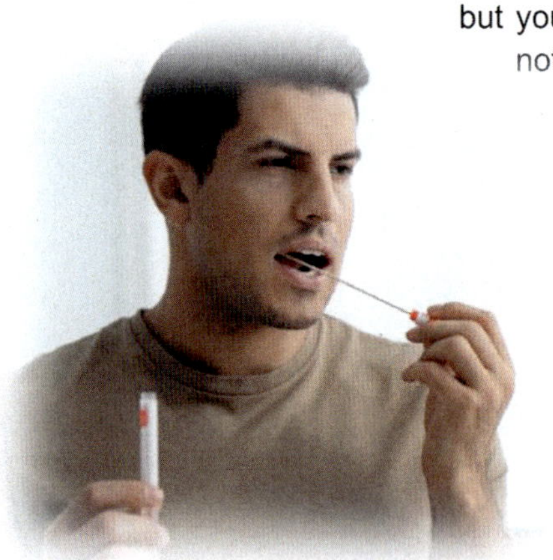

The test doesn't require a large sample of cells but you do need to be careful that there is nothing adhering to the inside of your mouth to avoid contaminating the sample.

A few weeks later, your report will be available for your clinician to interpret. The report is usually very detailed. Your clinician may give you an initial overview of its findings and then address the relevant SNPs sequentially over several visits.

Ideally, you would be guided to make certain dietary and lifestyle changes after each visit; you may also be recommended to take specific nutrigenomically-active supplements.

Do some research on the lab before you choose It's important to be aware that not all labs conducting nutrigenetic tests produce high quality analysis, so it's wise to do a little bit of research before you decide where to send your sample.[8] If the test does not require a clinician to provide the interpretation, you could very easily waste your money. That's because even if you can understand what the test means, the results are only useful if you know what changes to make to increase the expression of the *'lazy'* genes. This is where a trained clinician is essential.

Be cautious of surrogate gene tests In contrast to the lab test described above, there exists a surrogate test that is based on a questionnaire. You would answer a series of questions about your health status and when you tally up the ratings for each question, the report allegedly determines what weaknesses you are likely to have in about half a dozen genes. This is not a valid means of determining your nutrigenetic profile, so best to steer a wide berth.

CHAPTER 6

'Switches' that talk to your DNA

Just for a moment, imagine Christmas tree lights with about 200 tiny bulbs attached. The end of the cord is plugged into the power point on the wall. When you throw the switch, all 200 bulbs are illuminated at once.

It might surprise you to know that the cell's internal defence system works in much the same way. There are many different 'switches' within our cells but two in particular have profound effects on the way our cells work.

Meet Nrf2 A small protein known as Nrf2 is the equivalent of the Christmas lights' switch. But instead of lighting up lots of tiny bulbs, Nrf2 in the cell 'switches on' the cell's own defence system!9 In fact, this switch activates more than 200 or so different genes, all of which hold the DNA code for the many different aspects of cellular defence. Scientists call refer to these switches as transcription factors.

This is a very clever but logical strategy. How convenient to be able to activate families of related and supportive genes with the one switch! Nrf2 is a relative newcomer to our understanding of how cells protect themselves, having been known only since the mid-1990s.

Even though this was more than thirty years ago, it is a relatively short time when it comes to changing such a core concept that we've held onto for decades.

What's even more exciting than the discovery of Nrf2 itself is the fact that scientists have identified substances which can activate Nrf2. The most powerful known substance capable of activating Nrf2 is Sulforaphane which comes from vegetables of the Brassica family (part of the 'cruciferous' vegetable family [vii]).

Sulforaphane's potential as a therapeutic substance is so highly-regarded that it continues to be the subject of intense research in the hope that a patentable pharmaceutical medicine can be developed by modifying the natural molecule. Interestingly, it has not yet been possible to produce a modified sulforaphane[viii] which is any more powerful in its effect than Sulforaphane itself.

Meet NF-kB *(NF-kappa B)* Just as Nrf2 is a *transcription factor* in the cell's cytoplasm, so too is NF-kB. Where Nrf2's effect is to activate genes of the cell's defence system, NF-kB activates the genes which promote inflammation.[10]

We tend to think of inflammation as an undesirable phenomenon – and sometimes it is. You will recognize the effects of inflammation as being the red, hot, swollen appearance of an injured joint or effect of an insect bite. In both cases, *inflammation* is the necessary process the body uses to protect you against further damage.

Inflammation walls off the location from the rest of the body and stops the damaging stimulus from travelling further into other parts of the body. When you twist your ankle and it swells and feels painful, that inflammatory response forces you to immobilize the joint so that it can repair itself. It is most likely to be NF-kB which initiates this inflammatory process.

[vii] Cruciferous vegetables include the Brassica family, cabbage, broccoli, Brussels sprouts, wasabi, watercress and many more but only broccoli is a significant source of Sulforaphane.
[viii] Known as an 'analogue' when a molecule is similar to the native compound.

As the repair processes take over, NF-kB production slows and then stops; usually after a few days, the signs of inflammation have disappeared and early repair allows you to start to walk again, even though it may be a few weeks before full strength has been restored. That's the 'good' side of inflammation. However, in a person who has chronic arthritis of the joints, the inflammatory process doesn't shut down. Something has kept the NF-kB switch stuck in the *ON* position.

The triggers, as some form of irritant, which allow this to happen are not always easily identified. However, it is very clear that certain food molecules such as those found in deep-fried fatty foods don't just *'talk to the NF-kB gene'*, they shout loudly at it, telling it to keep the 'inflammation' genes switched on as they churn out large quantities of molecules called *inflammatory cytokines.*

Chronic inflammation (meaning that it continues over a long period) is a situation which underpins many diseases. Here are some examples:

Location of the Inflammation	Name of Condition
Inflammation of the joints	Arthritis
Inflammation of the airways (bronchi)	Asthma
Inflammation of the liver	Hepatitis
Inflammation of skin	Dermatitis
Inflammation of blood vessels	Vasculitis
Inflammation of the fine tubules of the kidney	Glomerulo-nephritis

Table 1: Inflammatory diseases by name and tissue type

Such chronic inflammation causes permanent damage to the associated tissues. These inflammatory conditions are often *'controlled'* medically by *anti-inflammatory* drugs. These drugs fall into two main families, the steroids and the NSAIDs (*Non-Steroidal Anti-Inflammatory Drugs*). Although both groups provide quite powerful reduction in the signs and symptoms of inflammation, they are responsible for a range of side effects, thereby restricting their long-term use. As with pharmaceuticals in general, these are just not sufficiently specific to target inflammation without producing *collateral damage* elsewhere. (*Remember the analogy of the sledge-hammer and the thumb tack in Chapter 5).*

One of the NSAIDs marketed as a 'breakthrough medicine' in inflammation control, *rofecoxib* and marketed as *Vioxx*, was withdrawn from sale in 2004 when it appeared to double the risk of heart attack in its users. Merck, the manufacturer settled a U.S. damages class action for $4.85 billion in 2007[ix]. Steroids similarly have long been known to produce a range of adverse effects when used for long periods. So, although pharmaceuticals such as these are a valuable part of crisis management, they are not really suitable for longer-term use.

So, what should one do when inflammation in one form or another seriously compromises day-to-day activities and enjoyment of life? Now, we've already seen that inflammation occurs in response to some type of *irritant* to the cells. This irritant can activate NF-kB in the cytoplasm. Once activated, NF-kB moves out of the cytoplasm and into the nucleus. Here, it lines itself up alongside the genes which code for the production of the *inflammatory cytokines.* Next thing, the cell starts churning out these cytokines which activate the inflammatory process. Very soon, the characteristic swelling, redness, heat, pain and consequent immobility seriously compromise quality of life.

Chronic inflammation shows itself in different types of diseases. In an individual predisposed genetically to asthma (inherited usually from the father's side), the inflammation appears as swelling of the bronchial

---

[ix] https://www.reuters.com/article/us-merck-vioxx-settlement-idUSL0929726620071109

tubes, affecting breathing. In those individuals predisposed to skin problems, the skin may begin to redden, itch and weep. Clearly, we need to know what the triggers are and how to limit their ability to keep NF-kB '*switched on'* when it appears to be unnecessary.

The good news is that we have answers to both problems. We do know to a large extent what the factors are that trigger the inflammatory process. And now Nutrigenomics has taught us that there are certain plant molecules[x] which can inhibit or '*switch off*' uncontrolled NF-kB.[11] Knowing how to regulate the process in both ways helps us to take control of diseases we may have thought we were '*stuck with*'.

Having the ability to *'turn down'* NF-kB to reduce the tendency for inflammation and *'turn up'* Nrf2 to help cells to protect themselves provides us with a powerful weapon against disease, whatever that disease may be named.

Having the ability to 'turn down' NF-kB to reduce the tendency for inflammation and 'turn up' Nrf2 to help cells to protect themselves provides us with a powerful weapon against disease, whatever that disease may be named.

As is becoming apparent, the ability to regulate cellular function is independent of the name of the disease. As we saw earlier in Table 1, the diseases listed as being inflammatory in nature all appear to be unrelated.

Typically, we consider diseases like asthma and arthritis to be completely unrelated but when we see them instead as different manifestations of uncontrolled inflammation in the cells, we see that there is a common link.

---

[x] To save you having to wait for the answer in Chapter 9, *Sulforaphane* has been shown to be a powerful inhibitor of NF-kB.

What this means is that when we look at health and sickness through the microscopic lens of the cell, we don't need to know the medical name of the condition. What we do need to know is the *abnormal process* leading to this condition.

Inflammation is one of the most common processes underlying common diseases. All chronic diseases appear to have an *inflammation* component. Knowing how to restore the natural balance to the cell's inflammatory processes puts us in the driver's seat. Pharmaceutical medicine seldom approaches illness in this way.

The next question we need to ask is, *"what are the triggers which lead to the inflammatory process initiated by NF-kB?"* And probably more importantly, *"what is the safest most effective way to switch off excessive production of NF-kB?"*

And as you guessed, *Nutrigenomics* can provide the answers!

CHAPTER SEVEN

Free Radicals & Antioxidants

A stroll through any supermarket will highlight many products with the term *'antioxidant'* prominently displayed on the label. Food marketers have been quick to pick up on consumer perception that 'antioxidants' are a desirable attribute of foods. This is a rather simplistic and incomplete view as we will soon see.

Free Radicals To understand the nature of an antioxidant, it is first necessary to describe a *free radical*[xi]. Without involving ourselves in too much chemistry, we can say that *free radicals* are molecules or atoms which have become unbalanced. To regain their balance, they attack other molecules, removing one of their electrons, thereby making the second molecule unbalanced. This process repeated over and over sets up a chain reaction. Whenever a molecule becomes an *unbalanced* free radical, it damages the part of the cell with which it is in contact. Naturally, cells try to avoid being exposed to uncontrolled and damaging free radical activity but when they do, they use antioxidants to neutralise potential damage.

Antioxidants Quite simply, antioxidants *'neutralise'* unbalanced free radicals, stopping the continuation of the chain reaction. We say that antioxidants *'quench'* free radicals. In that sense, antioxidants are essential tools for preventing uncontrolled cellular damage. *Appropriate* antioxidant reserves are one of the cornerstones of cellular defence, one of the themes of this book.

[xi] More correctly described as *Reactive Oxygen or Reactive Nitrogen Species* (ROS or RNS) but for familiarity, we will continue to use the term, *free radical.*

Many myths surround the concept of antioxidants and we can't explore all the issues here. However, it is important to know that the most powerful antioxidants are produced by the cells themselves. These cellular antioxidants are literally *millions of times more powerful* in their effect than those derived from foods or supplements. Vitamins C, E and beta-carotene, even at high doses have only a fraction of the antioxidant potential of the cell's own antioxidants.

The way a Vitamin C molecule quenches a free radical is like this; one Vitamin C molecule quenches just one or two radicals. In the process, the Vitamin C molecule becomes *oxidised* and can no longer function.[12]

Free radical **+ Vitamin C**	⟶	**Inactivated radical** **+ *Oxidised*** *Vitamin C*

Many of the foods being promoted to consumers as *antioxidant-rich* sources include pomegranate juice, grape juice, green tea and berries, especially blueberries. These foods contain a wide array of beneficial bioactive compounds but as antioxidants, their ability to quench free radicals is very limited, just as is Vitamin C.

Oxidative Stress When the extent of free radical activity in a cell is more than the available antioxidants can handle, the cell's reserves become so overwhelmed that we say the cell is subjected to *'Oxidative Stress'.*

When a cell is affected by oxidative stress, the resultant damage is likely to affect every part of it. This can include all the cell's critical functions; the energy-generating mitochondria, the protective membranes, key enzymes, the DNA within the genes, and more.

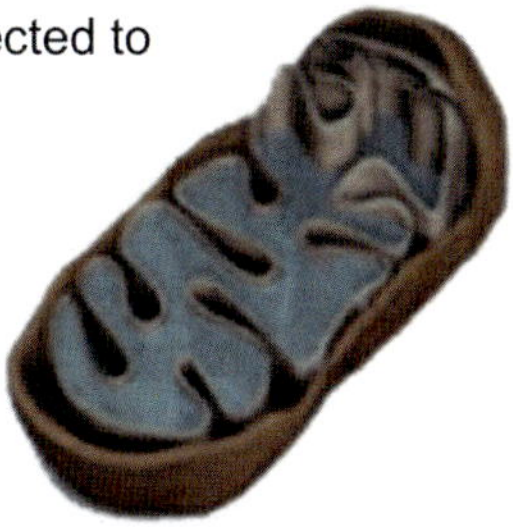

Figure 8 Typical Mitochondrion, known as the Powerhouse' of the Cell

Mitochondria and Fatigue Mitochondria, as we saw in Chapter 3, are the *'energy powerhouses'* of the cell. Consequently, loss of normal function of the mitochondria is likely to promote fatigue in the individual so affected. Not only do the mitochondria provide the energy that makes us feel bright and alert - but this same energy is required to drive every important function of the cell. If mitochondrial function is compromised, *EVERY OTHER FUNCTION OF THE CELL IS COMPROMISED!*

Not all free radical activity is harmful but if it overwhelms the cell's internal reserves and produces *oxidative stress*, widespread cell destruction will be the inevitable consequence. *Oxidative Stress* is known to underpin many diseases, including the major chronic diseases, heart disease, diabetes, asthma, cancer and arthritis.

The cell's own antioxidants which have the most profound effects on cell function are the following:

- **Primary Antioxidant Enzymes**
    - Superoxide dismutase (SOD)
    - Glutathione Peroxidase (GPx)
    - Catalase (Cat)
- **Glutathione**
- **Others**, some of which are enzymes and some which are not.

What is special about an Antioxidant Enzyme? An enzyme is a protein molecule that promotes a chemical process but doesn't get used up itself in the process. We describe it as a *catalyst.* Most of the chemical reactions which occur in cells require enzymes. So, when an *Antioxidant Enzyme* encounters a free radical, it quenches (*neutralises*) that free radical and then goes on to quench another and another and another.

The Antioxidant Enzymes literally quench *millions of free radicals per second* in this way and continue to do so over 3-4 days until the enzyme is broken down in the cell and replaced.[13]

Primary Antioxidants The pyramid diagram in Figure 9 shows that the greatest protection to the cell is offered by the three Antioxidant Enzymes, with *Superoxide dismutase* (or SOD) at the apex; these are known as the *Primary Antioxidant Enzymes.* As we saw earlier, the reason these enzymes are so powerful is that they can ***quench millions of free radicals per second.***

Secondary Antioxidants The Secondary and Intermediate Antioxidants (like Vitamins C and E) support the Primary Antioxidants but are so much more limited in their activity because one of these antioxidant molecules can quench only one or a few free radicals! Even taking megadoses[xii] of Vitamin C *(as many people do)* is a bit like tossing a glass of orange juice into the Pacific Ocean – the effect is minimal in comparison with that of the Antioxidant Enzymes.

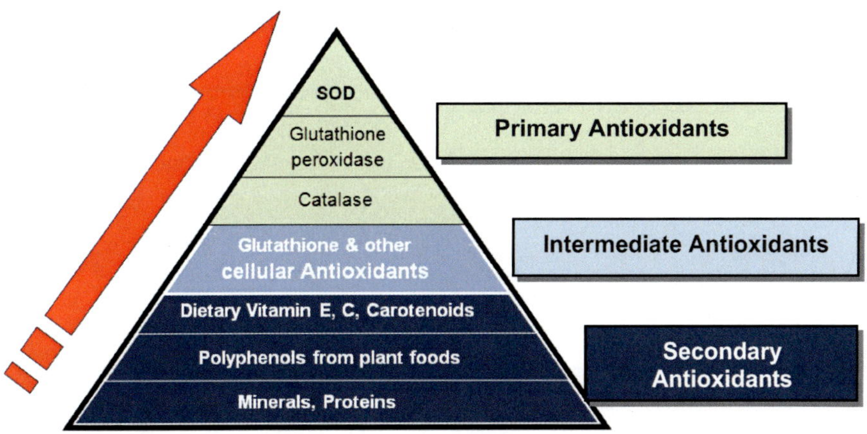

Figure 9: Increasingly Protective Effect with progress up the Pyramid

---

[xii] The US Recommended Daily Intake of Vitamin C is around 70-90 mg but varies for different countries. Many people take as much as 12,000 mg daily in the hope that this will confer greater antioxidant protection. However, there is no consistent clinical evidence to support this approach. As little as 500mg daily will saturate the cells and the remainder is excreted, unused. Learn more here from the US NIH Office of Dietary Supplements: https://ods.od.nih.gov/factsheets/VitaminC-HealthProfessional/#h2

Intermediate Antioxidants The intermediate category is made up of antioxidant compounds which are produced by the cells themselves. They are not *'catalytic'* in action like the Primary Antioxidants, so still directly quench just one or a few free radicals per antioxidant molecule. One of the better known of these is glutathione (*pr. Gloot-a-thigh-oan*). Glutathione is produced in large quantities by healthy cells to be sure it is ready and waiting when needed. The more potent Antioxidant Enzymes then take over, arriving at the scene a little later in response to cell signals to *turn up* their production.

Incidental Antioxidants The Pyramid diagram may give the impression that the secondary antioxidants are of little importance beside the Primary and Intermediate Antioxidants. However, all these substances have other very important roles to play in human cells. Vitamin C for example, is essential for normal function of skin, bones and teeth amongst other key functions but its antioxidant activity is not its strong point.

What this means is that all or most of the Secondary Antioxidants are largely *incidental antioxidants*; their primary function is something else. So when the supermarket shelves are displaying products claiming to contain antioxidants, these foods may have beneficial effects on human health – but they are unlikely to be particularly effective as antioxidants. Such foods, as we saw earlier, include green tea, berries, goji berries, grape juice, extra virgin olive oil, turmeric and so on.

ORAC Value You might have noticed food products which claim to have a high ORAC[xiii] value. This is a measurement which some food marketers like to use on their products as a way of inflating their apparent value in human health. The test is done in a laboratory with food samples in test tubes. What happens in the lab cannot be directly translated to what happens when the food is consumed. The inference is that the

---

[xiii] ORAC stands for **Oxygen Radial Absorption Capacity** and is a *test tube* measurement for determining a foods' ability to quench free radicals.

higher the ORAC value, the stronger the antioxidant potential of the food. This is not necessarily true for several reasons explained below.

Bioavailability[xiv] Many of the foods which rate high on the ORAC scale contain big bulky molecules called *polyphenols.* These molecules are so bulky that they don't easily slip through the cell's membranes. As a result, very few of the polyphenol molecules can enter the cell. The bioavailability of the polyphenols can be as low as 1%.[14]

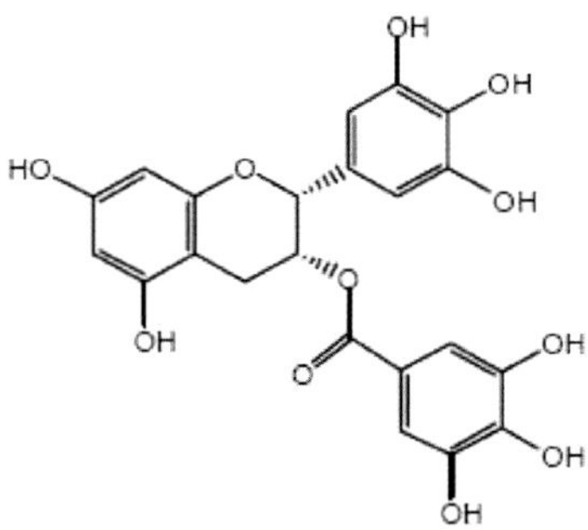

Impossibly large amounts need to be consumed for the substances to reach the cells in any quantity.

Figure 10: A 'bulky' Polyphenol molecule from green tea – known as EGCG. This bulk means that polyphenols are not readily absorbed through the cell's membrane. EGCG refers to Epigallo- Catechin Gallate.

As a consequence, these molecules contribute very little to the antioxidant capacity *within the cell or the bloodstream.* Where these polyphenol molecules do exert their antioxidant effect is in the digestive tract. Here the polyphenols are in *direct contact with the free radicals in the food itself.* Barbecued and processed meats and deep-fried foods of all kinds contain large quantities of free radicals and are known to contribute to various forms of cancer and other diseases.[15]

Because the bioavailability of the polyphenols is so low, it is not known whether the impressive *test tube* effects actually occur in human cells. It is unlikely that they do. In the test tube, many of the polyphenols appear

---

[xiv] Bioavailability is used to describe the percentage of a supplement taken by mouth which appears in the bloodstream, assuming that 100% of an intravenous dose of the same substance appears in the bloodstream.

to have nutrigenomic effects but how significant is that effect in our cells if we can't absorb very much of them?

The French Paradox The French are known to enjoy relatively low levels of cardiovascular disease in spite of the fact that they don't consume a particularly low-fat diet, as is usually recommended. Because it has been suggested that the polyphenol-rich red wine they consume with their main meals offsets their dietary fat, the term, *French Paradox* has been coined. *(Cheese, paté and butter are high fat foods.)*

Whether the red wine is the reason has not been proven beyond doubt but other scientists have suggested that there may be a protective effect from consuming various polyphenols with meals, especially at the same time as foods that contain known cancer-forming substances. An Israeli research group has shown that the polyphenols in one glass of red (but not white) wine is sufficient to completely quench the free radicals in an average meat kebab.[16]

Do you need to consume red wine to achieve this benefit? Now, I accept that you might *like* to consume red wine with every meal and if so, the evidence is that in moderation, this is beneficial. However, this may not suit everyone including children and those whose health is already compromised. There are many other polyphenol-rich choices and many of these are the same rich colour as red grapes. Foods such as hibiscus, pomegranate and beetroot, as well as most berries contain compounds similar to those in red wine. Significant health benefits have been attributed to these foods and continue to undergo investigation.

Green Tea and the health of Asians Some Asian populations but especially the Japanese have been able to achieve similar protection against cardiovascular disease by consuming polyphenol-rich green tea in significant quantities *with meals*.[17] And this is the key: *With Meals*. What the evidence seems to show overall is that the polyphenols act as antioxidants *in the digestive tract* and *not in the cells* - because too little actually gets into the cells to have an antioxidant effect. So, the message is that to get the most out of a polyphenol-containing food – or supplement – have it with the meal most likely to be a significant source of free radicals. That includes but is not limited to bacon, ham and other smoked foods, blackened foods of any kind such as barbecued or roasted foods, fried foods and even toasted bread.

So, whether you choose red wine, green tea, pomegranate juice, extra virgin olive oil, beetroot or any of the berries as good sources of polyphenols, ideally consume them regularly *with* a main meal.

Be wary of the Resveratrol hype! We can't leave this section without a word of caution. The polyphenol, *resveratrol* has been identified as a compound found in red wine and some claim that this is the reason for the *'French Paradox'*. Resveratrol has more recently been shown in yeast and animal studies to promote longevity. It appears to do this *nutrigenomically*, activating a gene known as *SIRT1.*

Even though there is absolutely *NO EVIDENCE* for any such effect in humans, supplement marketers have exploited the animal research to make resveratrol readily available as capsules or tablets. What the marketers omit to tell you, however is that:[18]

- The animals in the study (mice) consumed the human equivalent in resveratrol of about 1000 bottles red wine per day!
- 1000 bottles of red wine is about 75 capsules, each containing 100mg resveratrol. That would represent 7,500 mg daily.
- The only research in this field has been done on yeast, worms and mice where huge experimental doses were used.
- The longevity effect *only occurred when the animals were **started on resveratrol at birth***; no change from middle age.
- Resveratrol as a polyphenol has low bioavailability.[19]

There needs to be a little bit of scientist in each of us! Even if you are not trained as a scientist, always check that research used to support a product is conducted in humans at *practical* daily doses and not in animals using impossibly-large doses or worse still, in test tubes!

That is not to say that animal and *test tube* research is not valuable; it is an integral part of the progression towards our understanding of how a compound *might* behave in human systems. It just isn't enough on its own for us to draw useful conclusions about its potential value to us.

A quick word on Lipoic Acid and Coenzyme Q10 Two other important substances made in human cells exhibit antioxidant activity; these are *Lipoic Acid* and *Coenzyme Q10.* These substances have been reasonably-well researched in humans and are also available as supplements. Although both substances are promoted for their antioxidant activity, this is not their main function in the cell.

However, both substances as supplements have limited bioavailability; a standard oral dose of Coenzyme Q10 has a bioavailability of only 2-4%,[20] necessitating large doses to achieve a clinical response. The bioavailability of Lipoic Acid is better at around 30% but is still rather limited.[21] Note that *human cells make their own Lipoic Acid and CoQ10.*

What is the ideal Antioxidant? If we are to take advantage of the power of the Primary Antioxidants, the ideal supplement would have the nutrigenomic capacity to '*switch on'* or *'turn up'* the genes which code for the Antioxidant Enzymes as well as the other key cellular antioxidants, typified by Glutathione. But *only* when the cell needs them.

Do such nutrigenomic compounds exist and are they bioavailable? Before we go into detail, let's round out this section with a brief overview of the role of Glutathione, arguably the most important of the *non-enzyme* antioxidant compounds produced within your cells.[22]

Glutathione – essential for normal cellular function Glutathione is a rather remarkable and multi-functional small antioxidant molecule which is present abundantly in healthy cells but is easily depleted. It is essential in the process of detoxifying harmful substances.

As you might therefore expect, excessive consumption of alcohol readily depletes glutathione reserves. Similarly, cigarette smokers and those exposed to other forms of air pollution tend to have low glutathione reserves. This occurs because glutathione is consumed by the cells in trying to protect themselves against the harmful effects of the toxins associated with these two recreational drugs. Even the common analgesic, paracetamol (aka. *acetaminophen*), if taken to excess, will rapidly deplete glutathione reserves.

Individuals with oxidative stress-related diseases such as chronic asthma,[23] heart disease,[24] and diabetes[25] have also been shown to have abnormal cellular glutathione status. Typically, such individuals also show dysfunctional Antioxidant Enzyme activity in the three Primary Antioxidant Enzymes, especially *Superoxide dismutase* (SOD).

Can Glutathione be taken by mouth? Again, the supplement marketers have exploited the extensive body of science which describes the importance of glutathione in human cells and yes, glutathione supplements in various forms are available for purchase. Glutathione, which is made up of just three amino acids [xv] is readily digested by the secretions of the stomach.[26] What is the point of taking a preformed glutathione supplement which is quickly broken down into its constituents, with no glutathione remaining to be absorbed into the cells?

In the last decade or so, protected forms of glutathione have appeared on the market as supplements, preventing degradation by the secretions of the stomach. Although blood glutathione levels have been shown to

---

[xv] Amino acids are the 'building blocks' used to make proteins, assembled like a coiled string of beads. When a protein is digested, the amino acids are the end products.

increase when taking these forms, it is important to note that glutathione seldom acts on its own. It needs to perform its important biochemical tasks *in conjunction with other cellular molecules*. As we will see soon, our own cells are perfectly capable of making their own glutathione – *as and when they need it* – and in the amount that the cells require at that moment.

What about taking the *precursor* amino acids? One of the three amino acids which make up glutathione is said to be *rate-limiting.* This means that if it *(cysteine)* is in short supply, it reduces the overall production of glutathione in the cells. Attempts to supply extra cysteine haven't worked either as this amino acid is not bioavailable in this form. Another form of the amino acid, *N-Acetylcysteine* (NAC) has been found to act as a suitable precursor and can therefore be used to get more of the rate-limiting amino acid into the cell.

> *Important as the role of Glutathione is in the cell, increasing the Glutathione reserves with a supplement provides only a small part of what is required to enhance cellular defences.*

N-Acetylcysteine (NAC) however is not universally permitted for use as a supplement, even though it is used intravenously for paracetamol overdose in hospital emergency departments. In Australia where I live, the regulatory authority considers that there is insufficient evidence for its safety in humans to allow it to be used in an *over-the-counter* oral supplement.

Another limitation of NAC, even in those jurisdictions where it is permitted, is that glutathione is a member of a large '*supporting cast'* within the cell. Important as it is, it *is not the leading actor.* Glutathione is an essential *partner* to the Primary Antioxidant Enzymes, especially for *Glutathione peroxidase.* It is also an essential *partner* to the Detoxification Enzymes which are key elements in cellular defence.

What this means is that increasing the glutathione reserves plays only a small role in the activation of glutathione-associated pathways. What makes the real difference are the nutrigenomic compounds which can *'switch on'* the 200 or so cell- protective genes. Remember the Christmas tree lights analogy? Just one switch lights up 200 light bulbs all at once.

Why the antioxidant vitamins can do more harm than good. The new science of Nutrigenomics has completely changed the way Nutrition Science views supplementation with antioxidant vitamins. Although *high doses* of direct-acting antioxidant supplements like vitamins, C, E and beta-carotene have been popular for decades, there has been an uneasy and growing undercurrent of concern regarding their effects in human cells. Food-derived vitamins are not the issue; it is the high-dose supplements.

Theoretically, the antioxidant vitamins should be capable of quenching free radicals in cells. However, the evidence is conflicting, so that in some studies they have *no beneficial effect* and in other studies, they have been found to be harmful! [27]

Effect of beta-carotene on cancer prevention in smokers: In a large 1996 study,[28] smokers were given beta-carotene supplements to see if the development of lung cancer could be prevented; both smoking and cancer are associated with oxidative stress. The study had to be stopped early because the smokers on beta-carotene were developing lung cancer *faster* than the group taking the inactive placebo!

Effect of Vitamins C and E on benefits of exercise: Another study to investigate the effects of 1,000 mg of Vitamin C and 400 IU of Vitamin E in young exercising men showed that the antioxidant supplements actually *prevented the health-promoting effects of physical exercise*. This came as quite a surprise to the German research group who expected that the vitamins would provide an advantage.[29]

Instead, the metabolic benefits occurred in the placebo group with exercise only – but with no supplements. The exercise benefits were *completely negated* in the exercising group taking the vitamins!

What's going on? We now understand why such adverse effects might be occurring. *'Swamping'* the cells with excess antioxidant vitamins actually *'switches OFF'* Nrf2, hijacking the cell's major defences.[30]

The effect of Vitamin C supplements plus statin drugs: Another surprising outcome came from a 3-year study[31] where patients taking prescription statin drugs to reduce atherosclerosis *(build-up of cholesterol-like plaque in the artery wall)* were also given different doses of Vitamin C.

The patients were divided into five groups: Group 1, the placebo group had no supplemented vitamin C, whereas the remaining four groups took between 140 and 5,000 mg daily. Over the three years, the higher the Vitamin C dose, the greater was the thickening of the carotid artery in the neck. The effect on smokers was double that of the non-smokers. Very importantly, the researchers refer to the fact that *dietary vitamin C from food has been shown to have a protective effect* on the health of blood vessels – but it seems that *vitamin supplements* are another thing altogether.

Rethinking vitamin megadoses: Now, doesn't this *upset the apple cart* for the proponents of vitamin megadoses? Vitamins are absolutely essential to human health and do contribute to the *oxidative-antioxidant* balance of human cells – but they are ***NOT*** the cell's major means of doing so. There are now many studies that reaffirm what these three examples show – that it is wise to steer clear of synthetic isolated vitamin supplements, except for temporary use where a deficiency is evident.

There is nothing natural about taking excessively large doses of vitamins such as Vitamins A, C, E or beta-carotene. Such therapy is akin to using vitamins as pharmaceutical drugs. Human cells are not adapted to the presence of these vitamins in excess of the amount that can be manageably eaten in food.

More importantly, Vitamin C is synthetically manufactured in a laboratory and it might surprise you to know, no Vitamin C supplement has ***ever*** been anywhere near an orange ……. or any other fruit or vegetable!

CHAPTER EIGHT

Detoxification & Cellular Defence

Imagine the state of your car's performance if you never bothered to take it to the mechanic to be serviced. Failure to change the oil, grease various essential components and keep the running parts clean and tuned would result in sluggish performance – or worse! The cells of your body are no different. They need to be kept clean and have waste products removed regularly if they are to function at their peak year after year.

Most of us pay more attention to looking after our cars than we do our own bodies!

Unlike your car, your body doesn't need a mechanic to keep it in good running order; that's because you have chosen the highly-sophisticated *self-cleaning, self-tuning* model! The only thing you need to do is to regularly feed it what it needs most, move it appropriately and avoid over-stressing it. Depending on your individual DNA *'blueprint'*, you may or may not need to focus more conscientiously on certain aspects of its function.

Now, wouldn't you agree that many of us pay more attention to looking after our cars than we do our bodies – until something goes horribly wrong? And then, there's a quick trip to the GP, hoping that he or she can get rid of whatever sign or symptom sent you there. And as we saw in Chapter 1, what's going wrong *at the cellular level* is seldom corrected by mainstream medicine's pharmaceuticals.

Now, you're driving down the freeway in your under-serviced car and a red warning light on your dashboard flashes on. The red light is there for a reason – and in this case, probably to tell you the oil needs attention.

But you're far too busy to bother with the detective work, so you decide to pull over to the side of the road so that you can disconnect the bulb which has been annoyingly flashing red for the past 10 kilometres. Great – fixed the problem – no more annoying red light.

Now, isn't this a parallel situation to the use of a pharmaceutical drug when it is prescribed to get rid of a symptom? Does an anti-inflammatory fix the underlying cause of an inflamed joint, does an anti-histamine fix the underlying cause of the allergy and does an anti-hypertensive address the fundamental cause of the high blood pressure? Of course not; these prescriptions are just disconnecting the annoying red light bulbs, while the underlying cause continues to tick away silently in the background – for now! Eventually, your cells will be unable to cope and you find your health *suddenly* disappearing when a serious disease has been diagnosed. But none of this happened suddenly at all. We just chose to ignore the clues that may have been present for months, years or even decades!

Knowing how your cells defend themselves gives you the control to optimise their function and enhance your overall health and wellbeing. Understanding the cell's built-in *'spring-cleaning'* system is an excellent starting point. Whether you call it '*spring-cleaning'* or *'detoxification'* doesn't matter; the process is the same.

Do you remember that in Chapter 6 we looked at a *'switch'* in the cell known as Nrf2? Once activated, Nrf2 can move off into the nucleus to line itself up against the major genes which govern the cell's own defence system. When it is activated, it *switches on* or *turns up* all 200 or so genes at the same time. This defence system includes the genes of the cell's built-in detoxification system.

To simplify our understanding of the way cells protect themselves, we will consider a three-legged stool to explain the process. Of course, such a stool needs to have all three legs strong to remain steady. Before we get into the *nuts and bolts* of how cells detoxify waste materials, we should look at *WHY* a cell needs a Detoxification system.

What does the cell need to protect itself against? A live cell is continuously generating waste products from its many activities. These waste substances may be toxic chemicals - but they may also just represent 'clutter'. In any case, they need to be removed so that the cell's 'machinery' can continue to work efficiently.

One of the greatest threats to a cell's function is *oxidative stress.* This can occur when free radical activity exceeds the cell's antioxidant reserves. As we saw, free radicals can be present in food, especially in fried, overcooked and processed meats. Free radicals can also be generated by exposure to ionizing radiation, from the sun's UV rays to those of an X-ray. By far the greatest source of free radicals to which we are exposed is the huge quantity produced by our own cells!

How Superoxide Free Radical is formed Our cells require energy to function and a steady supply of this energy is produced in the cell's powerhouses – the mitochondria. In simplified fashion, the mitochondria '*burn'* the glucose from our food in the oxygen we breathe.

However, in the process, about 2-4% of the oxygen doesn't get used to produce energy. Instead, it is converted to a free radical known as *superoxide.* This might seem like a defect in the cell's function – but in fact, it is an essential part of the cell's signalling system.

***Superoxide dismutase* (SOD) to the rescue** Healthy cells are equipped to deal with the superoxide radical by generating the Primary Antioxidant Enzyme, *Superoxide dismutase* (or SOD).

SOD's job is to quench the excessive quantity of superoxide free radicals before they can set up chain reactions of free radical damage that bounce their way through the cells, wreaking havoc as they go. When free radical activity overwhelms the cell's ability to deal with it, *Oxidative Stress* results, potentially capable of causing damaging mutations in our genes.

There is now substantial evidence on chronic disease to show that the primary event which leads to all other effects is a state of oxidative stress.

This has been researched extensively in relation to Type2 diabetes,[32] asthma,[33] cerebro-[34] and cardiovascular disease, to name a few.

What is very clear from all these studies is that the closer we can get to dealing with the *CAUSE* of a condition, the better our chances of preventing it from getting out of control. Scientists use the term, *upstream factors* to refer to the earliest events in a disease. Knowing that free radicals set up chain reactions which magnify their effects as they go, it makes sense to try to get as far *upstream* as possible to stop widespread cellular damage.

> *When we use pharmaceuticals to deal with the symptoms of disease, we are only dealing with the 'downstream' effects. Working as far 'upstream' as possible gets us closest to the CAUSE of a disease.*

It should be clear then that when pharmaceuticals deal with the symptoms of a disease, they are typically dealing with the *downstream* effects. This is why it is so important that the cell keeps control of excessive free radical activity. As we age or are unwell, our cells become less efficient at producing these Antioxidant Enzymes when they are needed. In Chapter 10, we will look at some nutrigenomic mechanisms we can apply to enhance our ability to produce *Superoxide dismutase* at more youthful levels, even as we age.

How Diabetics are at increased Risk There is one more important point to make about the superoxide free radical. Most of the free radicals generated in the human cell are the result of burning glucose in oxygen to make energy! Types 2 Diabetes is a disease which is sweeping the globe and as more of us become progressively overweight and unfit, we are more prone to develop it. Why? Because as diabetics accumulate higher levels of glucose in some of their cells, the amount of glucose available to the mitochondria is higher. As a result, the 2-4% of oxygen which is normally converted to the superoxide radical is much greater in a diabetic than it is in a healthier person. Diabetics therefore produce substantially more superoxide than their cells can handle. Not only is a diabetic prone to the complications of diabetes itself but to *all the diseases* which are associated with oxidative stress in general.

As we will see in the following chapters, there are valuable *nutrigenomic* strategies we can use to support the improved lifestyle practices which are essential for optimum function.

So, in essence a cell primarily needs to protect itself from:

- ionising radiation
- chemical additives in processed foods
- heavy metals which enter the plant through the soil
- agricultural chemical residues which remain on the food
- inhaled environmental pollutants
- free radicals in inappropriately-cooked or processed food
- free radicals generated within the cell itself
- other metabolic breakdown products produced within the cell

Back to the Three-legged Stool Luckily, as owners of our own bodies we are not required to know and understand all the intricate processes a cell uses to do its own *'spring-cleaning'*. With a bit of basic care from us, the cell knows *exactly* what it needs to do!

The three legs of the *Detoxification Stool*

The three legs of the stool carry equal weight in ensuring that your cells are continuously being cleaned. Briefly, here they are:

1. **Antioxidant Status**, including glutathione – to *'neutralise'* cellular toxins or quench excessive free radicals.

2. **Detoxification mechanisms** – to break toxins down to harmless substances.
3. **Efflux pumps** – to pump toxic wastes out of the cell by activating 'shuttles' in the cell's membranes.

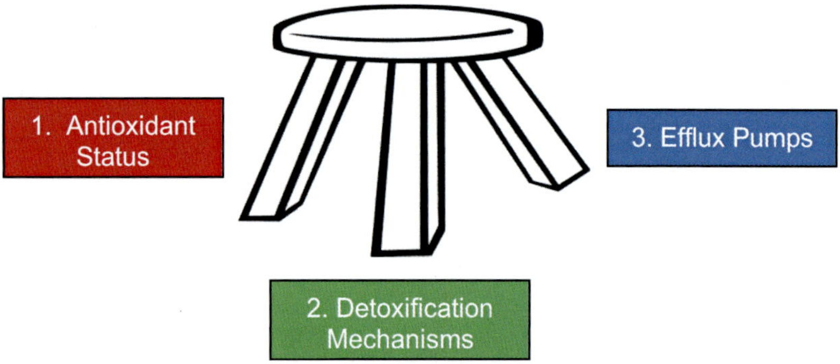

The good thing for us is that ***Nrf2 activates all three aspects*** of the Detoxification process. Therefore, we need to know the most effective *nutrigenomically-active* dietary compounds that will *turn up* Nrf2 and the production of not only our Antioxidant and Detoxification Enzymes but also our Efflux Pumps.

Here's how the Detoxification process works. Let's zero in on the actual process a cell uses in breaking down a toxin. Let's imagine that you have eaten some fresh spinach leaves that were grown on a farm.

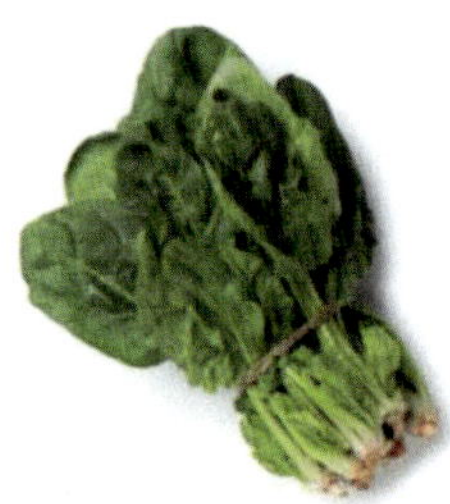

The spinach had been sprayed with pesticides so that the green spinach leaves arrived at the market in perfect condition. However, some of those chemicals weren't removed when you washed the vegetable before cooking it at home. After you've consumed the vegetable and it has been digested and the components absorbed into your bloodstream on the way to your cells, your cells recognise the presence of the toxic pesticide residue; they then *'crank up'* their detoxification machinery to break down those unwanted chemicals so that can be flushed out. Here's what they do.

Phase 1. The toxin is attacked by enzymes which belong to a group known as the *Cytochrome P450 family* (CYP450). CYP450 pulls the molecule to bits but can't totally inactivate it. However, it does what it can before passing it onto Phase 2, producing an intermediate compound and often large amounts of superoxide as well.

Phase 2. Phase 2 uses several Detoxification Enzymes which are known as *Phase 2 Detox Enzymes.* There are three main enzymes for detoxification (all with complicated chemical names). Two of these are important in our discussion, ***Glutathione-S-transferase*** (GST for short) and ***Quinone reductase***[xvi] (we'll call it QR to make things easy).

Let's say that the pesticide from our spinach required the GST enzyme for its second stage of detoxification. The intermediate compound is then presented to the GST enzyme, using glutathione as part of the process. After a few slick little chemical manoeuvres, what started out as a toxin capable of poisoning the cell is now released as a harmless water-soluble substance which can be readily flushed out.

Now there's just one potential problem here. When Phase 1 produced the partly degraded intermediate compound, sometimes that compound is more toxic than the pesticide that came from our spinach. Here's where a good reserve of antioxidants is so essential. The available antioxidants, (especially glutathione and SOD) are called upon to prevent a chain reaction of potentially damaging free radical activity.

If the antioxidant reserves are inadequate, this intermediate compound can severely damage the cell, including damage to the cell's DNA. This is one of the situations which sets the scene for the development of

---

[xvi] **Quinone reductase** is also described as **NAD(P)H:Quinone Oxidoreductase**

cancer cells, so it is critical that these Phase 1 intermediates are not being produced at a rate too great for Phase 2 or the associated antioxidants in the cell to accommodate.

***Superoxide dismutase* and Glutathione in key roles** Amongst the most important cellular antioxidants acting here are glutathione, *Superoxide dismutase* and the other Primary Antioxidant enzymes. These are then supported by less potent antioxidants from the food itself such as vitamin C, beta-carotene and other plant biomolecules.

Although the liver is the organ specialised to detoxify wastes, the process occurs in *every single cell* of the body, albeit to a lesser extent.

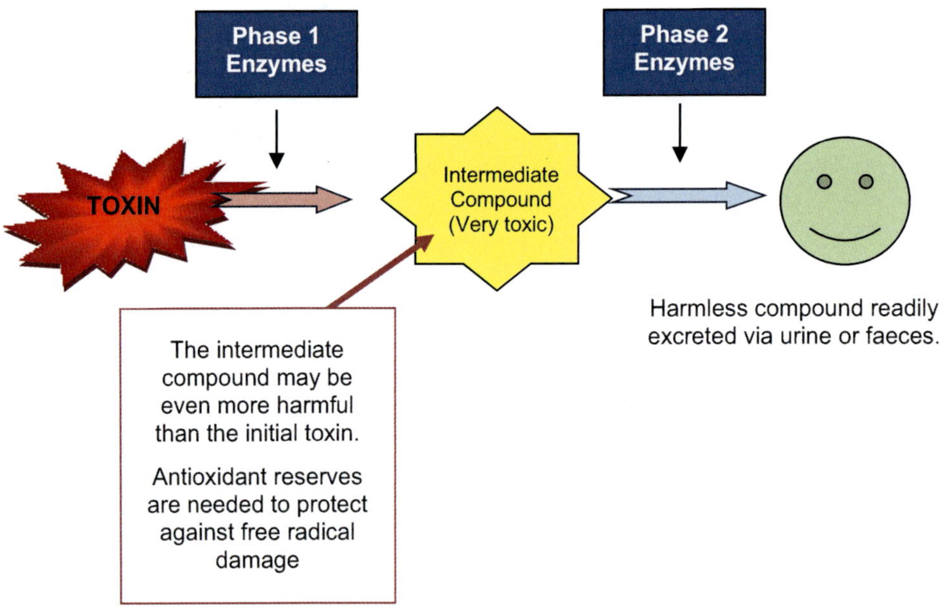

Figure11: The Detoxification Process

CHAPTER 9

Sulforaphane

One of the most extraordinary findings of our times is a small, sulfur-containing molecule, *Sulforaphane*, derived mainly from cruciferous vegetables such as broccoli. Although the plant doesn't actually *contain* any sulforaphane, it does contain two essential compounds (one of which is an enzyme). Both are needed to produce sulforaphane – but only when the conditions are right.

What makes sulforaphane so extraordinary is its ability to activate the cellular *'switch'* Nrf2, which, as we saw earlier, controls the 200 or so genes that are needed to produce key molecules of the cell's defence system.[35] In fact, sulforaphane is considered to be *the most powerful of the naturally-occurring substances* capable of doing this.[36] Better still, its high bioavailability of around 80% makes it a very practical supplement to the well-balanced daily diet.[37] As we have seen, much of the cell's ability to defend itself is by the activation of three key processes as shown.

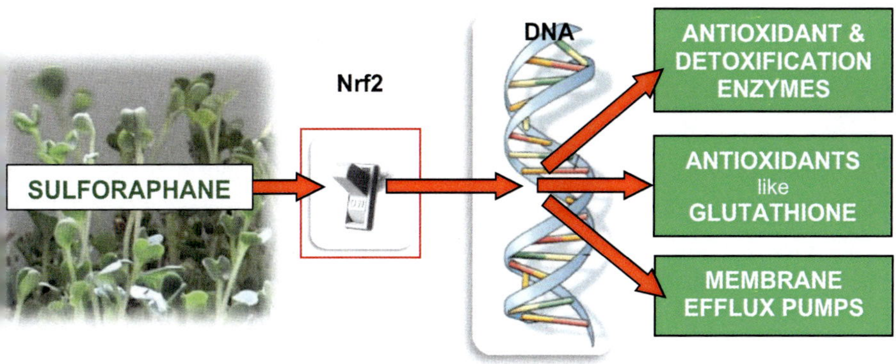

Fig. 12: How Sulforaphane 'talks to' your DNA, activating Cellular Defences

With these protective genes *'turned up'*, the cells operate more efficiently, energy is produced more readily, immune and inflammatory pathways are well-regulated and the cell's *'spring-cleaning'* processes remove waste materials before they have a chance to damage delicate cellular structures, including the DNA.[38] When *all 50 trillion of your cells* are working just as Nature intended, your entire body can operate at its peak. As we said at the outset, when your cells are healthy, *YOU* are healthy!

Status of Current Sulforaphane Research Much of the research conducted on sulforaphane in the last two decades has focused on its potential to prevent diseases for which mainstream medicine has few solutions; cancer,[39] heart disease,[40] asthma,[41] degenerative brain disorders,[42] gastric ulcers[43] autistic spectrum disorder[44] and type 2 diabetes[45,46] as the most notable. Each of these studies has been in the form of a clinical trial, the most meaningful way to determine if a food molecule will have beneficial effects when consumed by humans.

Sulforaphane has been used in hundreds of other laboratory and animal studies, continuing to add our knowledge of its many beneficial effects. There are now many research groups globally who are investigating different aspects of this remarkable nutrigenomic molecule.

This more recent research has also helped to explain why cruciferous vegetables more than other vegetable family, have been associated with prevention against disease in general, but especially against cancer.[47]

Diabetes and Sulforaphane Some of my own doctoral research focused on the potential for sulforaphane to prevent the life-threatening complications of type 2 diabetes and its severely damaging effects on the kidneys, nerves and blood vessels. There is already substantial evidence that the primary *upstream* event which leads to all other complications of diabetes is oxidative stress.[48] It seems the process is initiated by the *superoxide* radical and as we will see in the next chapter, a melon-derived nutrigenomic compound is capable of *turning up* the genes which code for the three *Antioxidant Enzymes*, led by *Superoxide dismutase* (SOD).

Where is sulforaphane found? It has been long known that broccoli doesn't contain any sulforaphane at all! Instead, the plant contains an *inactive precursor* compound known as *Glucoraphanin* in a sac within the plant cell *and an enzyme*, *myrosinase* in a separate sac. (*Figure 13*). Cutting or chewing the plant breaks the small sacs and a chemical reaction follows. This stimulates the myrosinase enzyme to convert the precursor compound, glucoraphanin to sulforaphane.

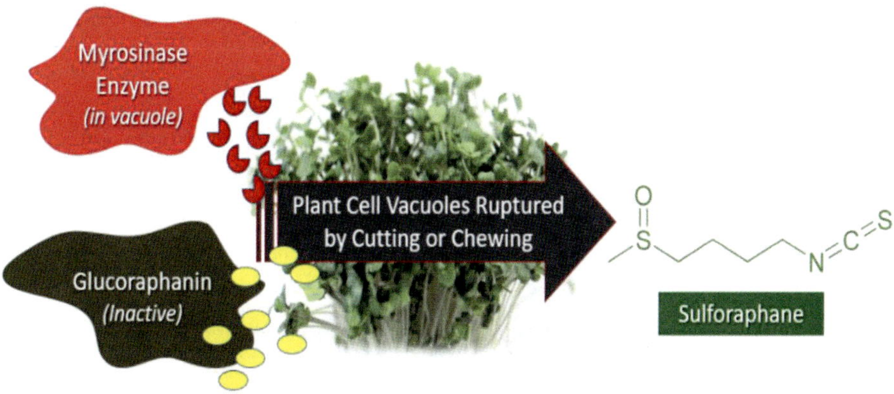

Fig. 13: Formation of Sulforaphane from Inactive Glucoraphanin

Other vegetables that need an enzyme to be active There are few plants that produce their bioactive molecule only when the plant cells are ruptured. All the cruciferous vegetables work like this – broccoli, cabbage, cauliflower, kale as common examples but the other vegetable family that is therapeutically inactive until chopped or chewed is garlic.

Garlic contains an inactive precursor, *alliin* which has no therapeutic nutrigenomic effect until its enzyme, *alliinase* converts it to the active (and odorous) molecule *allicin.* It is the *allicin* that gives garlic its health-promoting properties.

Interestingly, both the allicin from garlic and the sulforaphane from broccoli are produced by the plant as their own insecticide molecules. These molecules are toxic to a tiny insect – but therapeutic to large humans. The dose is what makes the difference!

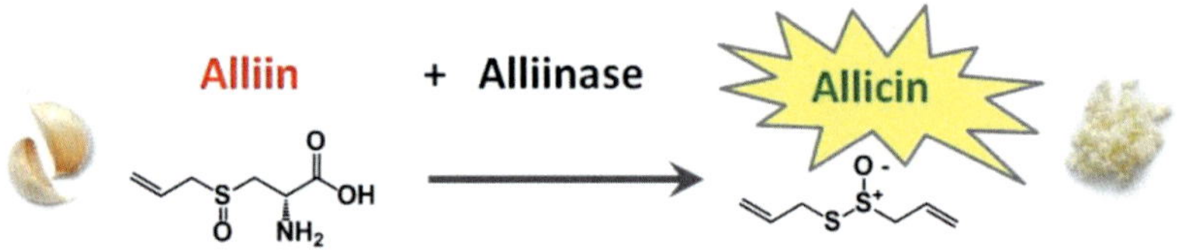

Figure 14: How an enzyme is essential for garlic to produce the beneficial allicin molecule. The alliin molecule in garlic is inert until acted upon by the alliinase enzyme. This is the same process that produces sulforaphane from the inert glucoraphanin when the myrosinase enzyme is activated by chopping or chewing. Note the similarity in the shapes of the allicin and sulforaphane molecules, compared to the bulky EGCG polyphenol molecule in green tea (Figure 10 on Page 41)

Cooking destroys the enzyme's activity Importantly, there is no nutrigenomic activity in broccoli or garlic if their respective enzymes are inactive. What this means is that the way we prepare these foods completely changes their beneficial properties.

Enzymes are found abundantly in both animal and plant cells and are absolutely essential for life. *But* - they are *very unstable molecules* - and are very sensitive to high temperatures and therefore, very easily destroyed by cooking. For this reason, we derive greater benefit from eating vegetables like broccoli, cauliflower, cabbage and garlic in their raw forms.

Chopping, grating and chewing activate the enzyme As soon as we cut, grate or chew these foods, the enzyme gets to work to produce the active molecule but its activity may remain for only 10-15 minutes. You could guess what happens if you buy coleslaw which had been made hours earlier. The bioactive molecule from cabbage (*sinigrin in this case, not sulforaphane)* is quickly formed but then rapidly degrades.

In broccoli, not only is the myrosinase enzyme easily destroyed but the sulforaphane molecule that is produced is also very unstable. This is why broccoli sprout supplements require a great deal of expertise if they are to retain their therapeutic effects when a person takes them.

How do I benefit from cooked broccoli vegetable? If cooking broccoli, cabbage, cauliflower and other crucifers destroys the myrosinase enzyme, how do I gain any benefit?

There is some research to show that the bacteria of the microbiome, a normal part of the human intestine, are capable of converting *glucoraphanin* to active *sulforaphane*; however, it turns out that the bacterial microflora are likely to convert as little as 8%-10% of the glucoraphanin.[49]

If you have recently had a course of antibiotics or generally have a gut condition known as dysbiosis, you may not produce any sulforaphane at all. You will still obtain the vitamins and minerals supplied by broccoli – but you will not obtain the protective Nrf2-activating effects.

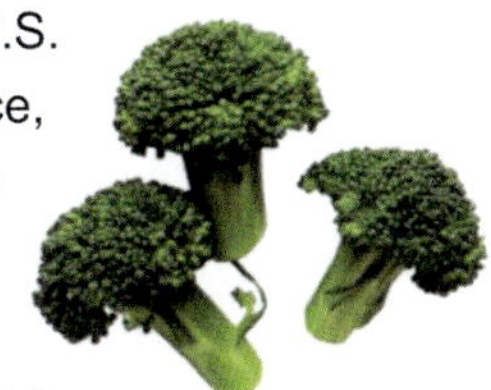

Vegetable vs Sprout A research group in the U.S. in the 1990s discovered that the precursor substance, glucoraphanin is found most abundantly in the tiny *sprouted seed* of the broccoli plant; in fact the sprouted seed contains 10-100 times more of this compound than the mature vegetable.[50] This finding makes it possible to obtain significant amounts of bioactive sulforaphane from only small quantities of broccoli sprouts.

As the science on this remarkable compound continues to unfold, it has become imperative that it be conveniently available as a functional food or nutraceutical supplement.

Growing broccoli sprouts It is possible for you to grow your own sprouts from broccoli seeds but such a process requires the time and a level of dedication few could muster on a regular basis.

Oddly enough, the fresh sprouts contain an inhibitor which partially *hijacks* the conversion from glucoraphanin to sulforaphane, instead producing an inactive sulforaphane *nitrile*.[51] Another important limitation to growing your own is that the amount of glucoraphanin in broccoli seed varies about 27-fold, so you might unknowingly buy seed with a very small amount of glucoraphanin.[52,53] You would never know because broccoli sprouting seed for consumers is never tested for its level of bioactives.

Powder or capsules for convenience

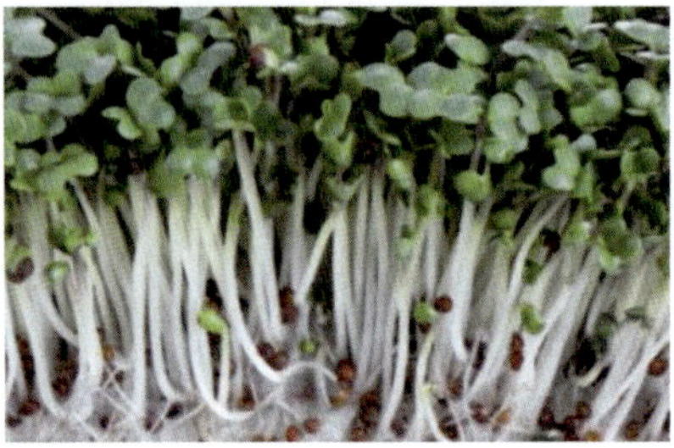

To obtain the consistent benefits of sulforaphane, the logical option is to take a powdered broccoli sprout product which can be consumed by stirring a teaspoon into water – or by taking myrosinase-active broccoli sprout capsules.

Perhaps surprisingly, the manufacturing process is not as easy in practice as it might seem. That's because the sprouts are very delicate and have to be dried carefully; at the same time, it is essential that the myrosinase enzyme is protected. The appearance of the powder cannot tell you whether or not it has retained its myrosinase; only a lab can do that!

Although industry is very experienced at producing many dried vegetable powders using the usual drying techniques, specialised technology is required to produce a broccoli sprout powder which can retain active myrosinase and be standardised for an optimal *Sulforaphane Yield*.

SPECIAL NOTE: Be very cautious about products which are simply made from *unsprouted* seeds. Broccoli seeds contain a chemical, *erucic acid* which is toxic to the heart - but fortunately disappears during sprouting.

Sulforaphane Yield vs Sulforaphane Potential Because the specialised technique required to produce a broccoli sprout powder with a consistently high *Sulforaphane Yield* is not widely-known, some of the products which have appeared on the market are of poor quality. When tested in the lab, many have been shown to have little or no myrosinase enzyme activity.

However, the label can be confusing because these products may claim a high glucoraphanin level. Others may also claim a numerical value for their 'Sulforaphane ***Potential***'. The 'Potential' as it turns out, is simply a calculated value based on a theoretical 100% conversion to sulforaphane ***if*** the product contained the enzyme.

Some products blatantly (or in ignorance) claim that their powder contains a defined amount of sulforaphane. As is already clear, the product *CANNOT* contain sulforaphane itself. The ideal product contains a high level of glucoraphanin along with active enzyme which should have been retained through careful processing. Once the powder is consumed, moisture activates the process of converting the glucoraphanin to bioactive sulforaphane.

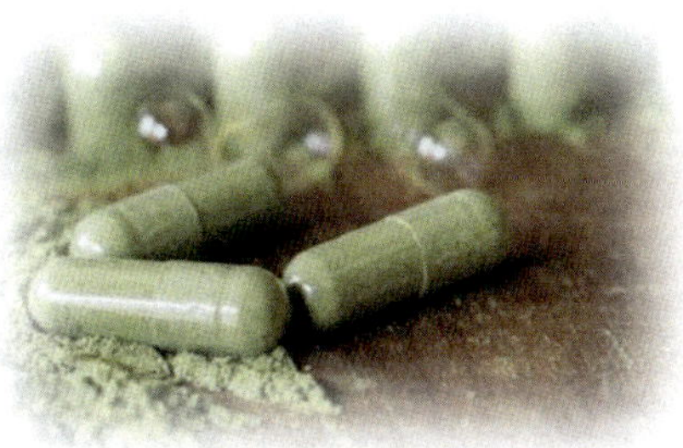

You can see how confusing it can be for the consumer to evaluate the worth of a particular product. However, once you do find a product which satisfies the criteria for bioactivity, it's surely worth making it an integral part of your day-to-day routine.

Healthier Ageing I've never been comfortable with the term, '*Anti-Ageing'* because surely there is no such thing! However, I do like the concept of *healthier* ageing because it is something over which we do have some control. Unfortunately, as we age, the cellular defence mechanisms become less efficient, making us more prone to illness. Even the *Master Switch* Nrf2 gets a bit 'rusty' and doesn't respond to the signals as efficiently as it did when we were younger.[54]

In Chapter 11, a completely new chapter in this edition, we explore a number of beneficial *healthy ageing* nutrigenomic effects which have emerged in the decade since I wrote the first edition of *"Switched On"*.

CHAPTER 10

Superoxide dismutase – coming to grips with Nature's *'antioxidants'*

At various intervals throughout earlier chapters, the Primary Antioxidant Enzyme, *Superoxide dismutase* (SOD) has been mentioned. In this chapter, we will see why this enzyme is so important and how it can be nutrigenomically activated. Following that, let's see how it compares with the familiar antioxidant vitamins.

SOD – why it is our PRIMARY antioxidant enzyme The main task of SOD is to quench (neutralise) excessive superoxide radicals soon after it is produced in the cell. Do you remember that 2-4% of the oxygen used in 'burning' glucose into energy in the mitochondria is converted to the superoxide radical? Although we tend to think of the superoxide radical as being harmful, there are several situations where it is essential to the function of healthy cells. Superoxide is only ever harmful when it is being produced at a rate that completely overwhelms the cell's own antioxidant capacity, especially the SOD enzyme whose job it is to keep it in check.

By a nasty twist of Nature, as we age, our cells tend to produce *more of the potentially damaging superoxide radical* while our overall antioxidant reserves progressively decline.[55] As a result, we are more likely to be in a state of *oxidative stress* as we age. This fact has significant implications for our state of health as the years advance.

Can we enhance levels of SOD? When the SOD enzyme was discovered in the late 1960s, it generated a great deal of excitement in the research world when the significance of this discovery was realised. Because of its relationship to the ageing process and the diseases associated with ageing, it wasn't long before it was considered to have *'anti-ageing'* possibilities, (even though we should say *'healthy ageing').*

Early research on injectable SOD The earliest research used a bovine source of SOD (marketed as Orgotein®) as a treatment for a range of diseases; osteoarthritis, rheumatoid arthritis and other inflammatory joint diseases. It was also shown to be effective as in reducing the side effects of radiotherapy, to name the most common.

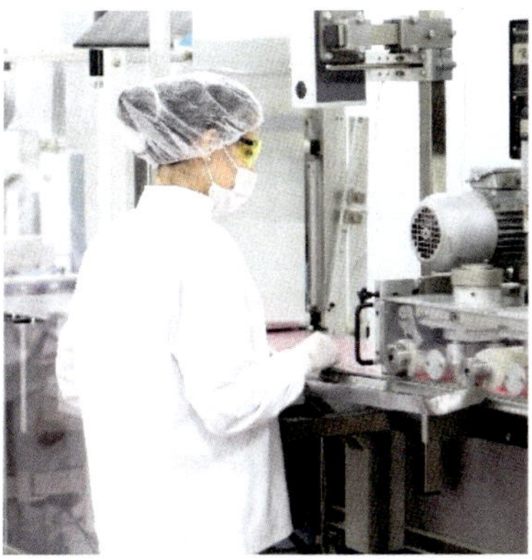

Orgotein®) was acknowledged as having *'potent anti-inflammatory activity with very low* toxicity'.[56] Orgotein, however, never realised its full potential because BSE or *'mad cow disease'* cast suspicion over any products of bovine origin and it was soon withdrawn from sale.

In spite of the very promising clinical responses, injectable SOD was not without its downside; the drug was both expensive and inconvenient, requiring daily shots. Its other serious limitation was that it provided SOD - but not its essential companion antioxidant enzymes, *Glutathione peroxidase* and *Catalase.*

A better option was needed When Orgotein® was injected into arthritic joints and other tissues where oxidative stress was dominant, only SOD was injected. Although SOD is essential for quenching millions of radical species per second, Nature produces companion molecules so that SOD works efficiently.

With Nutrigenomics, we are aiming to mimic Nature where genes tend to be *activated in groups* with related functions. When we activate SOD nutrigenomically, we also activate its companion antioxidant enzymes, *Glutathione peroxidase (GPx)* and *Catalase (Cat).* Better still, some other protective anti-inflammatory molecules are increased at the same time.[57]

Figure 15 shows how the potentially destructive superoxide radical can produce cell damage. But it also shows that when SOD is present, it converts superoxide into another radical, *hydrogen peroxide* which is also damaging. But when the two remaining primary enzymes are present, the *hydrogen peroxide* breaks down to harmless water and oxygen. This is why ***all three Antioxidant Enzymes*** must be present at the same time.

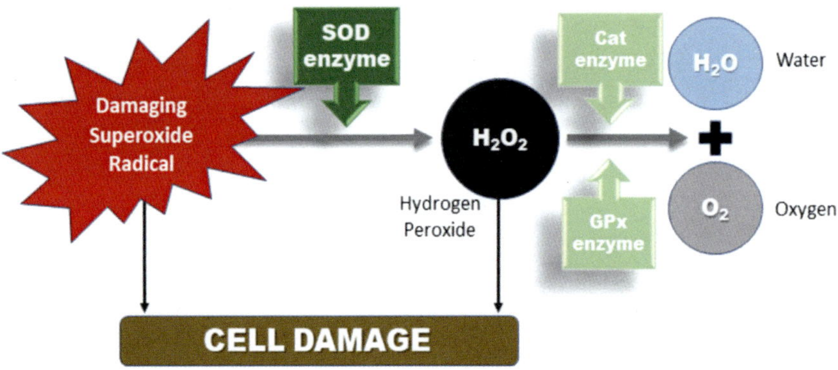

Figure 15: How toxic levels of superoxide radical are quenched when the three antioxidant enzymes are activated. The end products are nothing but water and oxygen. SOD – Superoxide dismutase; GPx – Glutathione peroxidase; Cat – Catalase.

SOD, the 'Lion Tamer' An easy way to consider the role of SOD in the cell is to see it as a Lion Tamer and superoxide the lion. As the lion tamer is in the circus ring cracking his whip, the lion behaves himself but as soon as the tamer loses control, the lion jumps the boundary and is out into the assembled crowd, wreaking havoc as he goes.

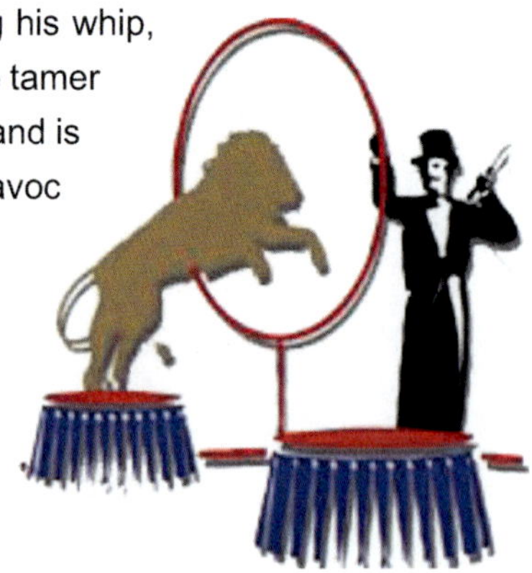

Such is the damage wrought by superoxide if it overwhelms SOD. As we age, we lose the ability to produce SOD as efficiently – a bit like having a very old lion tamer trying to keep control of a young willful lion!

Nutrigenomic activation of SOD So when bovine SOD was made unavailable by the 'mad cow' disease scare, it forced researchers to find another way to take advantage of this essential enzyme. A group of French scientists developed a melon-based SOD[58] using a patented process which allowed the enzyme to pass through the human digestive tract without being broken down[xvii].

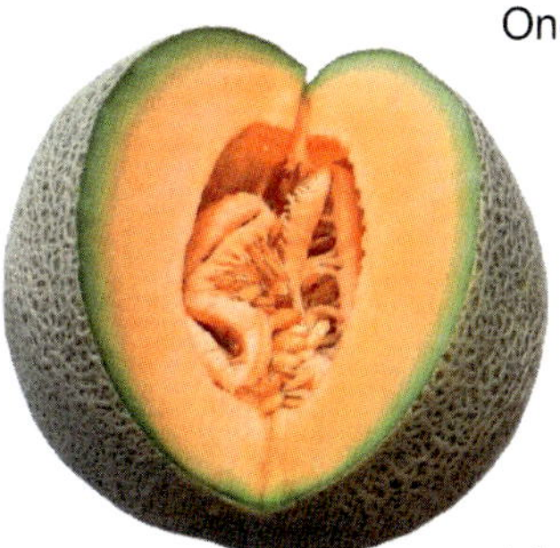

Once this form of SOD reaches the intestine, it exerts a *nutrigenomic* effect, *'turning up'* the genes which code for the antioxidant enzymes. Better still, it *'turns up'* all three antioxidant enzymes - *and not just SOD*. Quite serendipitously, this *nutrigenomic* response to the melon-derived SOD was superior to that shown by the bovine injectable!

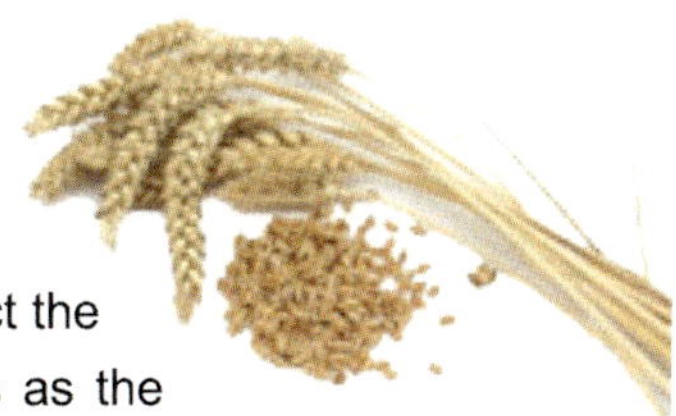

According to the patented process, a few milligrams of wheat-derived gliadin, about the size of a tiny breadcrumb, are combined with the melon extract to protect the SOD. At the same time, the gliadin acts as the nutrigenomic activator to *upregulate* SOD synthesis.

Clinical Trials demonstrating the value of *nutrigenomic* SOD There are two clinical trials which illustrate the enormous potential of this approach. In the first,[59] healthy male scuba divers were exposed to 100% oxygen at 2 ½ times atmospheric pressure for one hour. Such exposure is known to produce significant DNA damage, a real risk for deep sea divers. One half of the men had been pre-dosed with the melon-based SOD for two weeks, while the other group took an inactive identical-looking placebo capsule.

---

xvii Because food-derived SOD enzyme is a protein, it gets digested with other proteins in food. The patented process protected the enzyme from digestion.

When the DNA damage was analysed along with other markers of oxidative stress, *the group who took the supplement showed no damage at all.*

By comparison, tests on the placebo group showed the predictable DNA damage and other signs of oxidative damage. These findings were published in a respected peer-reviewed scientific journal in 2004.

Why not just use Vitamin C and E to protect the cells?
In an earlier chapter, we looked at the way in which dietary antioxidants (*the secondary antioxidants*) quench free radicals on a very limited basis.

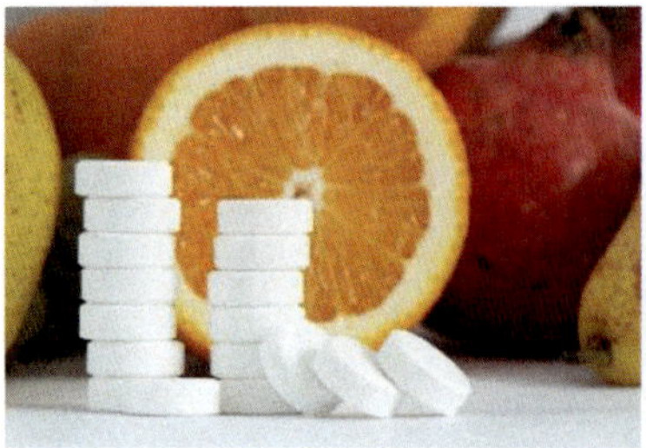

These vitamins lack the potency of enzyme antioxidants like SOD and its partners which literally *quench millions of free radicals per second.*

The following study illustrates the significance of this.

When antioxidant vitamins block protection This unrelated 2006 study[60] also used healthy men and exposed them in two groups to oxygen at 2 ½ times atmospheric pressure. The study group here took 500mg slow-release Vitamin C and 272 IU of Vitamin E for a month prior to exposure. The placebo group took *inactive* capsules.

The results of this study were remarkably different from the first; the *Vitamin C and E offered absolutely no prevention* against the oxidative damage caused by the hyperbaric oxygen. This study was also published in a respected, peer-reviewed journal. It's hard to argue with the evidence!

Cardiovascular Protection using melon-based SOD A similarly noteworthy three-year study[61] which was published in 2007 again illustrated the clinical significance of *nutrigenomically-active* SOD. This time, the study used individuals with pre-diabetic signs who had not been diagnosed with either frank diabetes or cardiovascular disease.

Such individuals will typically progress to significant levels of disease and could expect to be prescribed a range of pharmaceuticals designed to lower blood glucose, blood pressure and total cholesterol levels. All the participants in this study followed the Lyon Heart Diet *(a type of Mediterranean Diet).* Half took the melon-based SOD while the remainder took an identical placebo.

How the GliSODin melon SOD reduced artery thickening The study measured the usual markers of oxidative stress but they also used *carotid artery thickening*, a clinical measurement considered to be a gold standard[62] in assessing clinical change in a patient with heart disease.

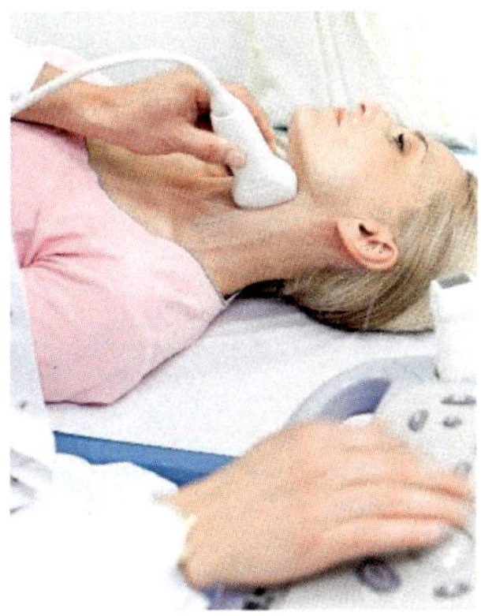

After two years, the group taking the SOD supplement showed *regression* of carotid thickening, whereas the placebo group continued to worsen. This is a remarkable result for a non-pharmaceutical compound. Typically, a *statin* drug would be prescribed to address abnormalities such as these in blood vessels. The *slowing* of arterial thickening is considered to be a positive result, especially in a condition which took years to develop.

The effect of a statin drug on atherosclerosis A two-year study similar in design to the one just described but which used a 40mg dose of a statin drug showed a *slowing* of arterial thickening but not *regression.*[63]

Typical of pharmaceuticals, statins are not sufficiently specific in their action to avoid adversely affecting other functions in the cell. The way statins affect cholesterol production in the cell is to block a key enzyme needed to produce it. However, this same enzyme is needed by the cell to produce its own Coenzyme Q10, an essential part of normal function of the mitochondria. This is why patients taking statins are often advised to take a Coenzyme Q10 supplement, even though the muscle pain that is a feature of statin therapy in about one-third of patients has not been shown to disappear with the addition of Coenzyme Q10.

Antioxidant Vitamins in Cardiovascular Disease Regardless of the theory, several large-scale trials involving many thousands of subjects have failed to show any benefit in prevention of cardiovascular disease by non-nutrigenomic antioxidant vitamins. Perhaps surprisingly, some studies showed that higher-dose vitamin E (more than 400 IU per day) might even be harmful!

The 5 points worth remembering: As you may have noticed, some of the biochemistry here is rather complex and it is not necessary to delve into it any further. But there are a few highlights that are worth remembering if we are to take advantage of the nutrigenomic message for the benefit of our own health.

Let's focus on these 5 key points:

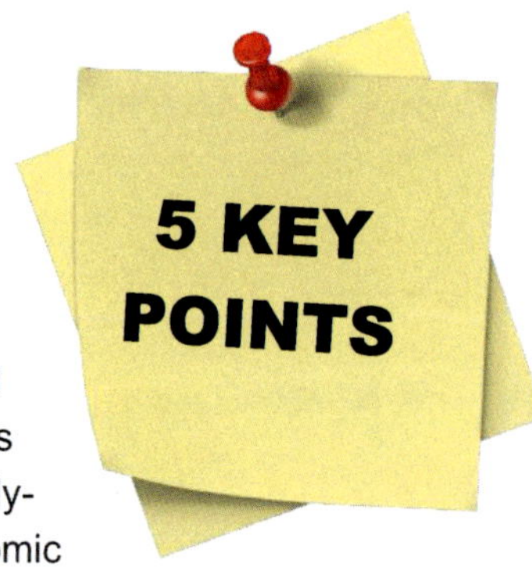

1. **A new model for antioxidants** Our thinking on 'antioxidants' has changed dramatically in the last few decades. Our own cells make very powerful antioxidant and detoxification *enzymes* which are essential components of the defence mechanisms of our cells. We can use nutrigenomically-active foods or select nutrigenomic supplements to promote this effect.
2. **Cells activate their own defences** Cells activate these powerful defences by detecting 'danger' or 'stress' signals from their immediate environment.
3. **Free radicals are no longer the 'bad guys'** Free radicals – or reactive oxygen species – are the *signals* that *'switch on'* a couple of hundred genes of the cellular defence system.
4. **Avoid synthetic antioxidant vitamins** Synthetic antioxidant vitamins like Vitamins A, C, E and beta-carotene have very little

ability to quench radical species when compared with the enzymes we make ourselves.

5. **Nature doesn't use megadoses – nor should we.** Megadoses of antioxidant vitamins as well as the popular supplement *N-acetyl cysteine* (NAC) block the signals cells use to activate their own defences. We can obtain all we need from a healthy lifestyle with well-balanced plant-rich diet, mimicking the principles of Nature.

If you are inclined to read scientific papers, here is a useful 2010 discussion from well-respected academics working in this field. *Antioxidants: Molecules, Medicines, and Myths by Gutteridge and Halliwell.*[64] The paper explains why the direct-acting antioxidants to which we have become so accustomed, simply cannot do what we expect them to do when taken as supplements.

How do I use this information for my own health? In Chapter 6, we saw the power of activating Nrf2 to '*turn up*' several hundred of the genes that govern the defensive processes of our cells. Naturally, we will want to do this – but how?

Nature's way is to employ something as simple as good food, exercise and adequate rest. There is nothing new about such recommendations which you have known all your life. But the reality is that most of us somehow haven't managed to make these three a regular part of our routines.

However, we can 'cheat' a little by taking supplements of two of the most powerful nutrigenomically-active plant concentrates. You already know about sulforaphane from Chapter 9 and now in this chapter, we have introduced a melon-gliadin extract known as GliSODin®.

I never recommend using supplements as an alternative to a healthy lifestyle but including specific foods or concentrates with measurable nutrigenomic activity can enhance the function of each and every one of our cells.

CHAPTER 11

Nutrigenomics and the Ageing Process

The ageing process is an inevitability none of us can escape, even though we may spend a small fortune in trying! It's easy to see that some of us age better than others, leading us to ask what we can do to be one of those who seems to *age gracefully,* remaining physically healthy and free of age-related chronic disease.

At intervals throughout earlier chapters, the Primary Antioxidant Enzyme, *Superoxide dismutase* (SOD) has been mentioned; in the last chapter, we highlighted its role in cardiovascular health and illustrated its superiority to the antioxidant vitamins.

Let's now expand on its role in the ageing process. But before we do, we need to keep in mind that what we have already learned about Nrf2's ability to activate disease-protective genes is equally important in healthy ageing.

SOD and protection from the sun It is well-known that excessive exposure to the sun's ultraviolet radiation is highly damaging to our skin, leading to unattractive dark patches on the skin, dryness, deep wrinkling and roughened texture. Although this cannot be completely prevented, there are ways to minimise these effects.

French Scientists target these processes naturally In France where melon-derived SOD was developed, dermatologists have been researching its effect on protecting the skin against sun exposure. As we saw in Chapter 7, radiation generates reactive species, or *free radicals.* Not only is excessive sun exposure responsible for sun burn but over time, it alters the texture and resilience of the skin.

The formation of compounds known as ***A**dvanced **G**lycation **E**nd products,* conveniently called AGEs is a characteristic of ageing skin.[65] AGEs develop when sugar molecules such as glucose attach themselves to proteins, therefore reducing the normal function of the proteins. AGEs are responsible for cross-linking the protein chains in the major proteins of the skin, *collagen* and *elastin*, so that these proteins lose their ability to stretch and contract normally. Clearly, approaches to limit the formation of AGEs in skin are a key to healthy ageing.

The melon-based SOD has been investigated for its effect in recovery from sunburn across a range of skin types.[66] When pre-dosed for two weeks before exposure to UV radiation, the treated groups showed significantly faster recovery than the untreated. It was also noted that in the fairer more sensitive skin types, up to *nine times* more UV exposure was tolerated in the treated group. Research in this area continues.

Superoxide and the Skin Ageing Process The superoxide radical is produced at various locations in the cell but one of the most abundant sources is from an enzyme family known as NAD(P)H Oxidase; usually abbreviated to NOX.

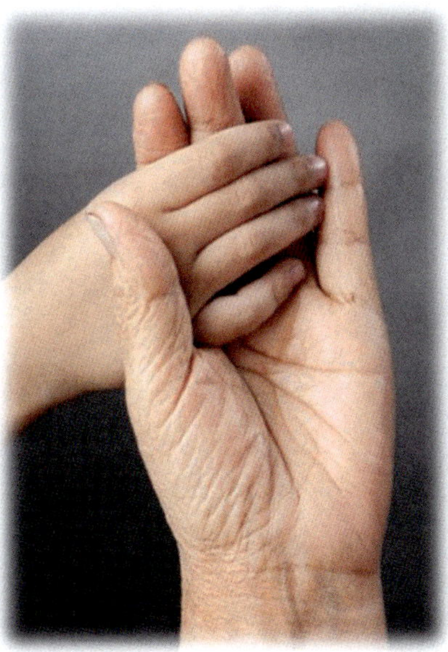

Interestingly, some of the members of the NOX family are only produced as we age, appearing at around age 30 and peaking at about 55 in women and 65 in men.

Because the levels of NOX are directly correlated with skin damage regardless of exposure to the sun, it is generally considered that it is the excessive superoxide radical which could be responsible.

SOD, as we have seen, has been shown to reduce levels of this skin-damaging superoxide, so nutrigenomic inducers of SOD such as the melon-derived form become the logical choice for helping to protect the skin against premature ageing.

Nutrigenomics and the Immune System A fascinating 2008 study on aged animals showed that sulforaphane restored Nrf2 activity to the levels of much younger animals. Abnormalities in the immune system commonly accompany old age and this study showed that using sulforaphane increased glutathione levels in these animals. Moreover, their immune function returned to normal and signs of skin allergy cleared. This has rather exciting possibilities for future research but whether the same response will occur in humans is yet to be seen.[67]

Other Theories

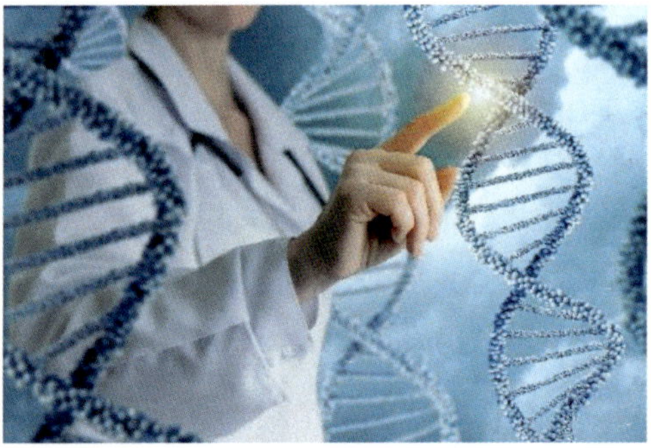

Some researchers have hypothesised that blocking NOX activity in the skin might be a way of reducing the skin ageing process. Attempts to find compounds which do this are under investigation. Some of the substances found to block the NOX enzyme are the statins, salicin, apocynin, Coenzyme Q10, green tea and an extract from the daffodil bulb.[68,69] As we saw in Chapter 7, both Coenzyme Q10 and the green tea polyphenols have very poor bioavailability, so may not be ideal for this purpose, even though they are promoted as such.

Furthermore, Coenzyme Q10 in high doses may also block the signalling required to activate Nrf2. Whether blocking the NOX enzyme is effective remains to be seen and at this stage of the research, it is probably too early to know.

Should we even try to block an enzyme? Of more concern is whether it is a good strategy to block a naturally-occurring enzyme. We do not yet know whether this approach is safe because there is insufficient evidence. As we saw earlier, the *statin* drugs used to block the cholesterol-producing enzymes are not without side effects because this enzyme is associated with other desirable functions within the cell. Blocking a naturally-occurring cellular enzyme would seem to fly in the face of Nature's inbuilt processes.

Nutrigenomics already allows us to work *with Nature* to restore the cell's Antioxidant Enzymes to levels more closely associated with younger cells. Blocking an enzyme may have effects we can't yet predict and why artificially block an enzyme which produces superoxide when SOD is Nature's built-in mechanism for handling excessive free radical production? Better still, published peer-reviewed research confirms the clinical value of one approach but not of the other!

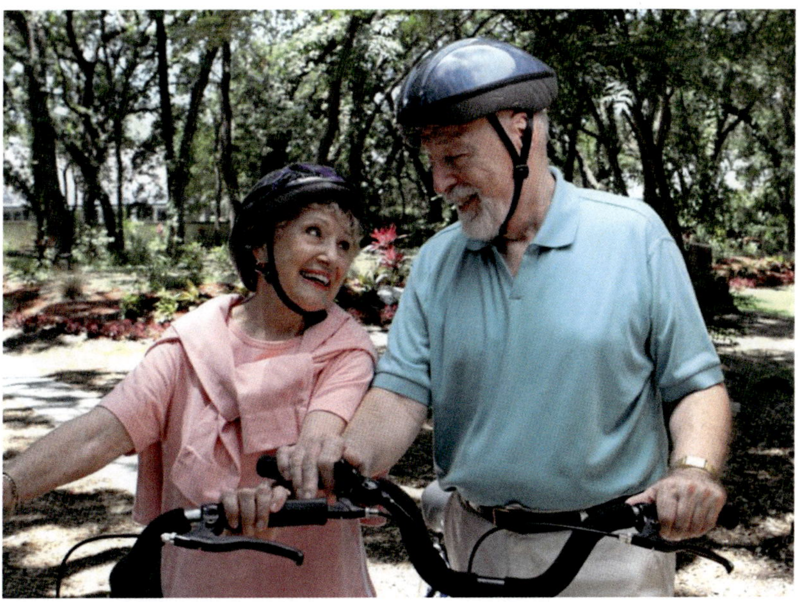

CHAPTER 12

How Clinicians Use Sulforaphane

Because sulforaphane is both highly-bioavailable and highly potent in its ability to upregulate protective genes and downregulate pro-inflammatory genes, its investigation has become a very popular research topic, especially for those researchers with an interest in clinical solutions for disease prevention and treatment.

Figure 16 shows how rapidly the number of peer-reviewed annual publications has grown since 1992 but has especially accelerated since the first edition of *"Switched On"* came off the press in 2010.

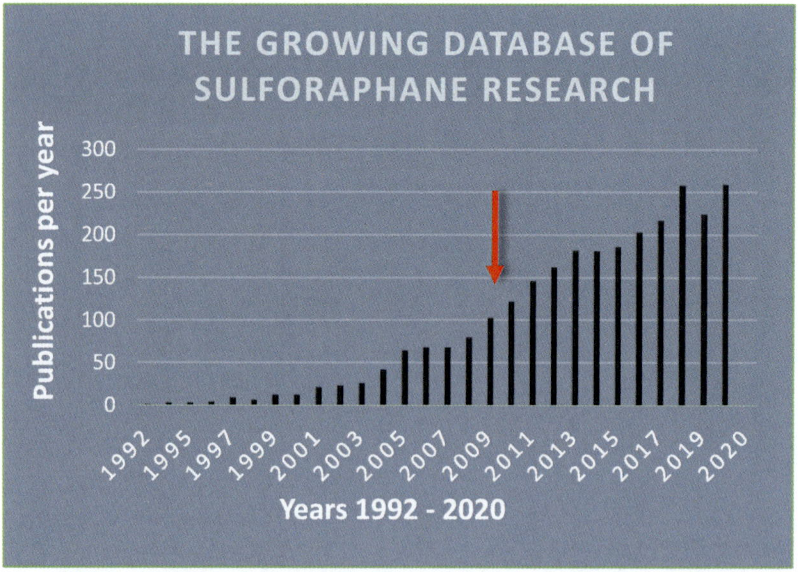

Figure 16: Rapidly-accelerating research into all aspects of sulforaphane

Highlights of Sulforaphane Research Scientists investigating molecules that may have therapeutic potential perform their research in three fundamental ways. If they suspect a plant molecule may have therapeutic effects, they start in the lab by trying to understand how the molecule works.

1. **Lab Bench Studies:** This often means adding a measured amount of the molecule to animal cells in a petri dish and then observing what happens. To gain an understanding of how the molecule works in human systems can take years. The very first studies on broccoli sprouts in the early 1990s were aimed at finding out why broccoli and other cruciferous vegetables could be protective against the development of cancer.

   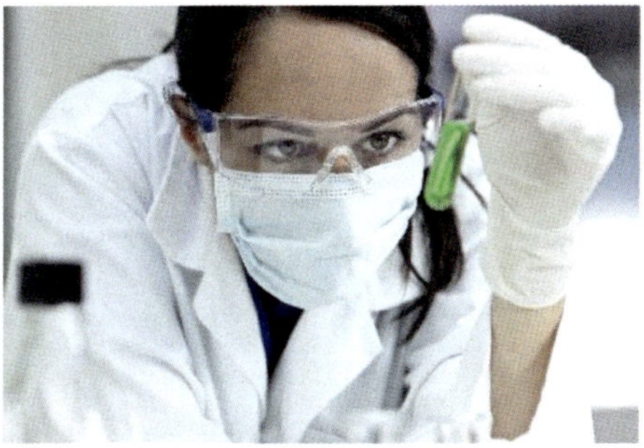

   Researchers performed lab studies from which they discovered that sulforaphane was very capable of increasing the activity of particular detoxification enzymes in the liver.[50] They showed that one of these enzymes *Quinone reductase* (Chapter 8) when activated, was able to prevent mutations in the DNA of cells.

2. **Animal Studies:** Once scientists gain an understanding as to how the molecule works in cells, the next step is to study its effects in animals. This allows scientists to see if it actually works in a live situation in helping to relieve symptoms of a disease.

   Depression is one of the most common psychiatric disorders in humans, so the need for safe and effective solutions is imperative. A Japanese research group used mice to investigate depression-like behaviour (yes, mice can get '*down in the dumps*' too). Knowing that depressive states in humans are closely-related to inflammation and aware that sulforaphane has anti-inflammatory effects, the Japanese scientists designed a study in inflammation-affected mice.

They pre-treated the animals by injecting them with stabilised sulforaphane, comparing their results with a second group of mice that had not been given the sulforaphane.[70,71]

Their results showed that sulforaphane had indeed blocked the increase in inflammatory cytokines in the brain regions related to mood. They concluded that there was enough evidence from the animal study that human studies were warranted.

Although there is not, at the time of writing, a clinical trial using sulforaphane to treat depression, there is a trial in progress to investigate its potential effectiveness as an adjunctive treatment in Bipolar Disorder.[72] The trial, "*The efficacy and safety of sulforaphane as an adjuvant in the treatment of bipolar depressive disorder*" began in mid-2020.

3. Human Clinical Trials

It is not uncommon that when a lab study or an animal study is modified for a human clinical trial, the same encouraging results are not always seen. This was the case for the early resveratrol 'anti-aging' studies where the increased longevity seen in worms and fruit flies was never seen when human studies were conducted. Sulforaphane, by contrast, has demonstrated some very favourable results in human clinical trials.

A range of human trials using sulforaphane have been conducted over the last few years, investigating conditions that include *autism, asthma, Type 2 diabetes, Helicobacter pylori infection of the stomach* and others. You will find more information about these studies in Table 2 below. What is really useful is that the doses used in the studies can be readily achieved with a good quality myrosinase-active whole broccoli sprout supplement.

Table 2: Clinical Trials using sulforaphane in various human conditions

CONDITION	DAILY DOSE of Sulforaphane	AUTHOR	YEAR
SUPPLEMENT STANDARDISED FOR SULFORAPHANE DOSE			
Autism	9-14 mg	Singh et al.[44]	2014
Asthma	18 mg	Brown et al.[41]	2015
Nasal Allergic Response	18 mg	Heber et al.[73]	2014
Chronic Obstructive Lung Disease	19 mg	Riedl et al.[74]	2009
Helicobacter pylori infection	30 mg	Yanaka et al.[75]	2009
Detoxification (atmospheric pollution)	35 mg	Egner et al.[76]	2011
Type 2 diabetes	40 mg	Bahadoran et al.[77,78]	2012
Prostate – PSA doubling time	60 mg	Cipolla et al.[79]	2015
FRESH BROCCOLI SPROUTS *			
Helicobacter pylori infection	14-56 grams fresh sprouts	Galan et al.[80]	2006
Inflammation markers in overweight	30 grams fresh sprouts	Lopez-Chillon[81]	2018
Gastric Mucosal Repair	70 grams fresh sprouts (183 mg glucoraphanin)	Yanaka A. [82]	2011
Metabolic Syndrome	100 grams fresh sprouts	Murashima et al.[83]	2004
GLUCORAPHANIN AS MYROSINASE-INACTIVE BROCCOLI 'EXTRACT'			
No prevention with 6 pills branded 'extract'	180 mg glucoraphanin – not sulforaphane	Atwell et al.[84]	2015
SULFORAPHANE SUPPLEMENT – NULL RESPONSE TRIAL			
Helicobacter pylori infection	2 mg	Chang et al.[85]	2015

CHAPTER 13

How the G.E.M.M. Protocol embraces Nature's Principles

As we have already seen in the pages of this book, modern medicine has trained us to expect *a pill for every ill*. This is easy therapy for us as patients and we have certainly come to expect this level of convenience. If only human cells were so amenable to this approach when the illnesses are complex.

One of the problems with this approach is that, although we are happy when we see the symptoms disappear, we typically don't address the cause(s). Ticking away inside the cells of our bodies are disease-promoting processes and if we don't deal with these promptly, it may be only a matter of time before another symptom appears. The result? Often another pharmaceutical prescription – or worse, the need for surgery.

In the decade since the first edition of *'Switched On',* I became progressively more aware that the principles of nutrigenomics as outlined in this book needed to be simplified. They also had to be available in a form that anyone could easily incorporate into his or her personal health management programme.

The acronym G.E.M.M. is derived from *Gut Ecology and Metabolic Modulation*. There is a growing awareness that many human ills begin in the gut and indeed, a large body of scientific evidence supports this. This is one of the foundation principles that underpins the way we implement the G.E.M.M. Protocol.

What is not well-known is that around 80% of our immune function resides just under the cells lining the gut.[86] Because the cells lining the gut and large numbers of immune cells are in close contact with each other, the

G.E.M.M Protocol adopts strategies to address the relationship between both types of cells.

The sciences behind G.E.M.M. When I developed G.E.M.M, I realised that it would have to embrace many different biological sciences if it was to create a link between the gut, its complex underlying immune network and the different body organs and systems.

Even though we say the science on which G.E.M.M. is based is complex, we also say *the implementation is simple*. What makes the science so complex is that it has had to integrate several branches of biology; as a consequence, G.E.M.M. clinicians are trained to embrace the key elements of these typically unfamiliar scientific disciplines.

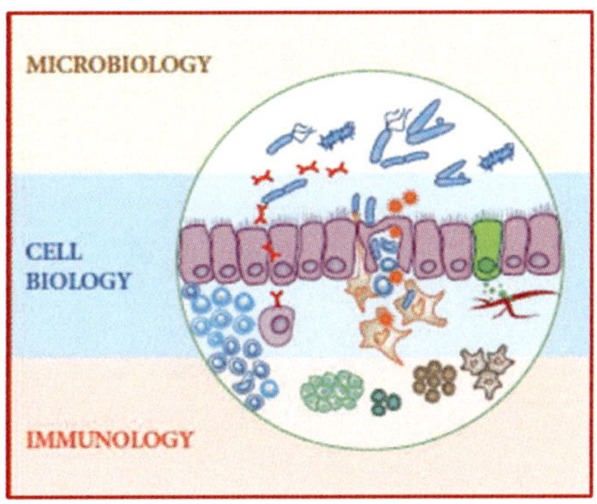

Figure 17: The 3-compartment Gut Ecosystem, the Microbiome, the Gut Epithelium (lining cells) and the underlying Immune Network.

1. **Cell Biology** describes much of what is happening in the gut lining cells, known as the epithelial cells. We refer to these as *Mission Control* of the gut ecosystem, because if we can restore their function to normal, or at least close to normal, lots of other issues will correct themselves.
2. **Immunology** is the science that describes the function of the immune system, shown in Figure 17 to directly underlie the gut epithelium.
3. **Microbiology** is the science that explains the function of the microbiota – the *bugs* - that inhabit the gut. Where we once thought that all microbes living within our bodies were harmful, we now know that populations of *friendly* microbes are essential for good health.

4. **Nutrigenomics and Biochemistry** underpin all the above functions, because both human cells and microbes are responsive to the signals produced by food and environmental molecules.

From complex science to an easy-to-implement protocol After reading literally thousands of scientific papers across several scientific disciplines, my greatest challenge lay in taking such complicated science and working out how to integrate all the information into a complete system that could be easily followed by anyone.

G.E.M.M., as you will see later, aims to follow as closely as possible the principles of Nature. This makes it notably different from the many current popular approaches to gut health.

Popular treatments for gut issues

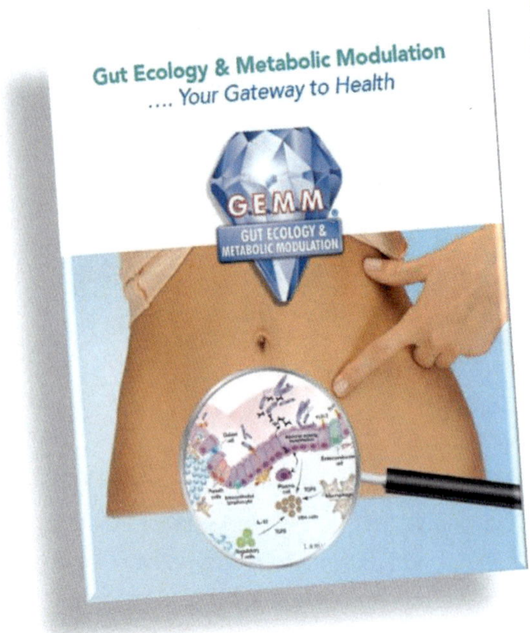

Gut health has become a popular topic for the many people who suffer a range of distressing symptoms; some conditions are mild but increasingly we see that many people suffer severe symptoms that are longstanding.

Untreated, some gut problems can be life-threatening, so should always be taken very seriously and investigated thoroughly to rule out the more serious conditions.

Irritable Bowel Syndrome – an umbrella term The term, *Irritable Bowel Syndrome* is something of an umbrella diagnosis for a whole collection of symptoms. The term can encompass bloating and discomfort with or without eating; it can mean frequent bouts of diarrhoea, persistent constipation – or even alternating bouts of both.

In others, the discomfort is in the upper digestive tract, leading to embarrassing belching and acid reflux, both of which may affect appetite. Medically, there are many pharmaceutical options but these seldom ever correct the underlying cause of the problem. In some cases, medications that relieve stomach discomfort by reducing the release of acid needed for protein digestion can lead to other complications that may affect the microbial population further down the digestive tract.

Do we need so many 'labels'? Some of these gut conditions have been given their own *labels* such as *'Leaky Gut Syndrome'* and *'Small Intestine Bacterial Overgrowth (SIBO)'*. A variation of SIBO has been labelled as *SIFO to* describe a similar condition which is thought to be due to fungal overgrowth.

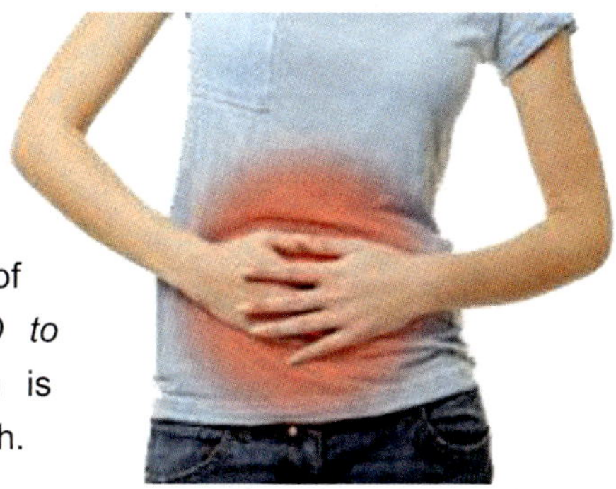

These labels are not typically recognised by mainstream medicine, although there are some doctors who do acknowledge and treat them as sub-categories of gastrointestinal disorder.

Anti-microbials and Probiotics as Therapy? Medical and non-medical clinicians who treat these conditions recommend both pharmaceutical and non-pharmaceutical therapies. Commonly prescribed are supplements with anti-microbial properties, designed to kill specific microbial species of the gut.

Even though such anti-microbials may kill the harmful pathogen, they are not specific to that organism and therefore destroy an unknown number of the 'friendly' microbes of the gut; this approach is more than likely to further destabilise the microbiota of the gut ecosystem.

Anti-microbial therapy is typically followed by recommendation of a range of probiotic supplements, even though we know there is limited ability of probiotic bacteria to take up residence in the gut. For decades, clinicians and consumers alike have assumed that the organisms in probiotic supplements would colonise the gut. What has emerged is that we have had very poor understanding of this topic and many of our old assumptions are now in doubt.[87]

Probiotics as therapeutics have been actively researched for decades and many probiotic organisms can influence the gut environment as they pass through. As such, they are useful in relieving many unpleasant gut symptoms.

Without the ability to colonise the gut, the effect is short-lived unless other steps are taken to correct the gut environment as a whole.

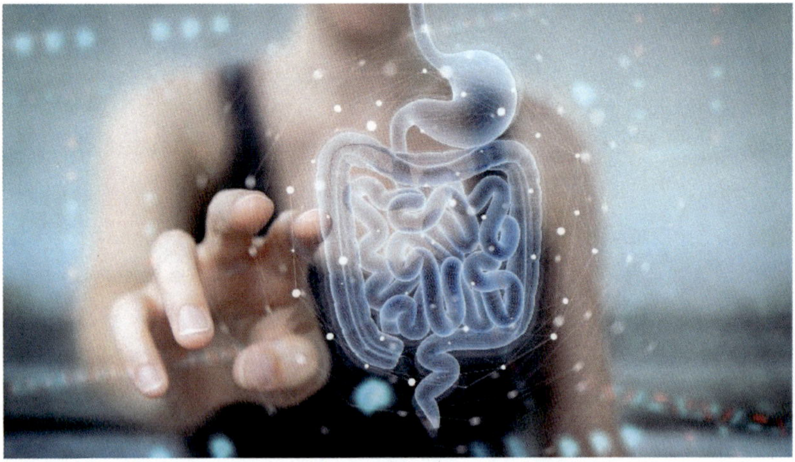

Modern Science to the Rescue From a G.E.M.M. perspective, these variations in normal gut dysfunction do not require their own labels; nor do they need extensive – *or expensive* - testing. When a clinician employs the core principles that normalise imbalances in redox, inflammation, detoxification and energy production within cells, normal function returns to the gut epithelium and its underlying immune network. We discussed these principles in earlier chapters. Normal balanced function in the gut-immune interface is known as *homeostasis.* In G.E.M.M., sulforaphane plays a key role in restoring homeostasis.

When gut-immune homeostasis is re-established, numerous symptoms disappear. Perhaps surprisingly, many foods that have once been reactive can now be tolerated. This is because many food intolerances occur because the gut epithelial lining cells are highly-inflamed; this chronic inflammatory state is then exacerbated by certain foods.

By eliminating the inflammation and oxidative stress from the gut ecosystem, food molecules are no longer reactive; in this way, G.E.M.M. can correct food intolerances.

Looking to Mother Nature for Answers We know that humans have existed on this planet for millennia, and without modern medicine. This begs the question; *How has Mother Nature sustained human life for so long without pharmaceuticals*?"

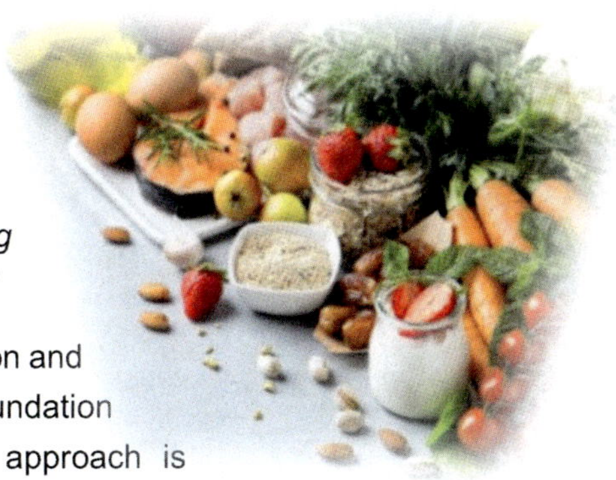

This is a very good question and the answer forms the foundation on which the G.E.M.M. approach is based.

This is not say that we don't need life-saving medicines; we very often do. However, they are usually better left until *after we have tried safer options* that are more aligned with the way Nature solves such problems.

How is G.E.M.M. different? After working for decades with thousands of patients with all types of conditions, I realised that clinicians in Nutritional Medicine were prescribing too many synthetic vitamin and mineral supplements. Although the human genome had become accustomed over millennia to vitamins and minerals naturally found in food, that was not necessarily the same as exposing the genome to synthetic supplemental forms, all of which contain other excipient ingredients as part of the tableting or encapsulating process.

After delving into phytochemical research, I was soon armed with an understanding of Nutrigenomics, a science which completely changed the way I was to think about nutritional therapy. I reasoned that if I could work out how best to mimic the processes used in Nature, clinicians could use this information to prevent and treat disease.

And so G.E.M.M. was born, rich in scientific evidence, its foundation anchored in the principles of Nature and translated into the context of a 21st century lifestyle. Keen to make the G.E.M.M. Protocol more widely available, I now teach other clinicians how to take advantage of this remarkably effective but gentle approach.

The Gut-Immune-Metabolism-Disease Link As we saw earlier, around 80% of our immune system resides just below the layer of cells lining our digestive tract (or gut). Perhaps surprisingly, if you are prone to infections of any kind, your gut will be involved. Even more interesting is the fact that the connection between the gut and the immune cells, *the gut-immune interface,* is linked to every other organ of the body.

Figure 18 illustrates the intricacies of the *Gut-Brain Axis*, one of the better-known examples of the many internal links between the gut and our many organ systems.

G.E.M.M. provides not only a way to target problems in your immune system – but G.E.M.M. uses the gut-immune interface as the gateway for dealing with conditions in the rest of the body. When this gateway is not working as it should, all sort of things in your body chemistry will start to go wrong – joints may ache, blood glucose levels may not be properly regulated, moods can be unstable, hormones may become unbalanced and skin rashes can appear seemingly out of nowhere. The systems that are affected is determined partly by the genetic blueprint we were born with and partly by our lifestyle and environment.

The name *Gut Ecology & Metabolic Modulation* tells us that by restoring the gut to normal, we can correct problems in our metabolism. Interestingly, it is claimed that the Father of Modern Medicine, Hippocrates who was born in 460 BC, said *that 'all disease begins in the gut'.*

Although technically this may not apply to *ALL* disease, it has taken us 2000 years to appreciate his knowledge and wisdom!

What we didn't know until relatively recently is that the 'friendly' bacteria and other microbes living in the healthy digestive tract are absolutely essential for the immune system to function normally.

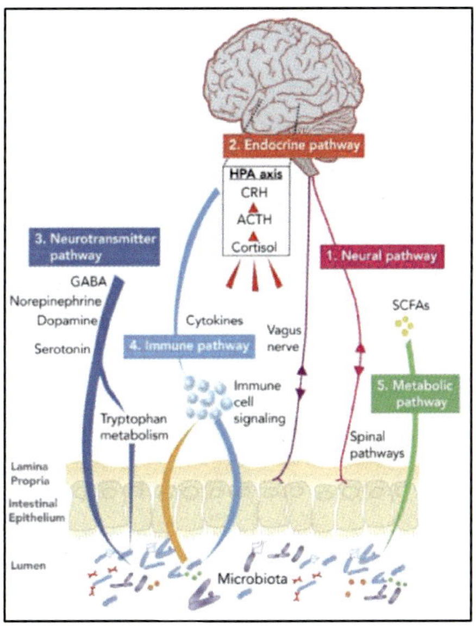

Figure 18: The Gut-Brain Axis as an example of the complex signalling that occurs between the Gut-Immune Interface and the brain.

(Please refer to page 102 for a larger version of Figure 18.)

Food – much more than vitamins and minerals Clinicians practising Nutritional Medicine have known for decades that what we eat has an enormous impact on our health and well-being. In those countries where the people live long and healthy lives, the food they eat and the lifestyles they lead have been directly linked time and again to their good health.

Traditional Mediterranean diets are a good example of this and even in Melbourne, Australia where elderly Greeks continue to grow and eat their own vegetables, their lifestyles have been shown to play an important role in their health as they age. Not only are they eating healthy home-grown fruits and vegetables but they are also obtaining fresh air, sunshine, exercise and a sense of purpose, all of which are essential contributors to good health. From a nutrigenomic standpoint, such lifestyle factors also activate the cellular *'switches'* that lead to the expression of hundreds of protective genes.

How Food 'talks to' our DNA Modern Nutrition Science has shown us that food provides us with so much more than proteins, fats, carbohydrates, vitamins and minerals. Plant foods in particular are a rich source of thousands of compounds we call *phytochemicals* (*phyto-* means *plant*) and it is these that contribute to our health in so many important ways. The polyphenols from red wine and green tea as discussed in Chapter 7 are examples of what we call *phytochemicals;* so too is sulforaphane.

It turns out these phytochemicals send powerful messages to the DNA in our cells, activating the defence mechanisms that protect our cells from harm. On the other hand, overly-processed refined foods send messages that increase the activity of inflammation-causing mechanisms.

Not only do these phytochemicals contribute greatly to nutrigenomic activation within our cells but they also provide a valuable source of food for the microbes that live 'happily' within our bodies. When I wrote the first edition of "Switched On" in 2010, very little was known about the important links between the gut and the rest of the body.

This new scientific focus on the gut and its underlying immune network has enabled me to combine the core principles of nutrigenomics with what we now know about the role of the gut and its underlying immune network.

G.E.M.M. captures the very essence of Nutrigenomic Medicine and envelopes it in 21st century science, reaffirming the mechanisms that were unknown to the many generations of ancestors who walked this planet, surviving and thriving according to the principles of Nature.

G.E.M.M. is founded on an approach that seeks to mimic the principles of Nature – but in the context of life in the 21st century. As such, G.E.M.M. is so much more than a means of addressing gut health, even though it targets the Gut-Immune interface as a first step in addressing whole body physiology to restore and maintain good health.

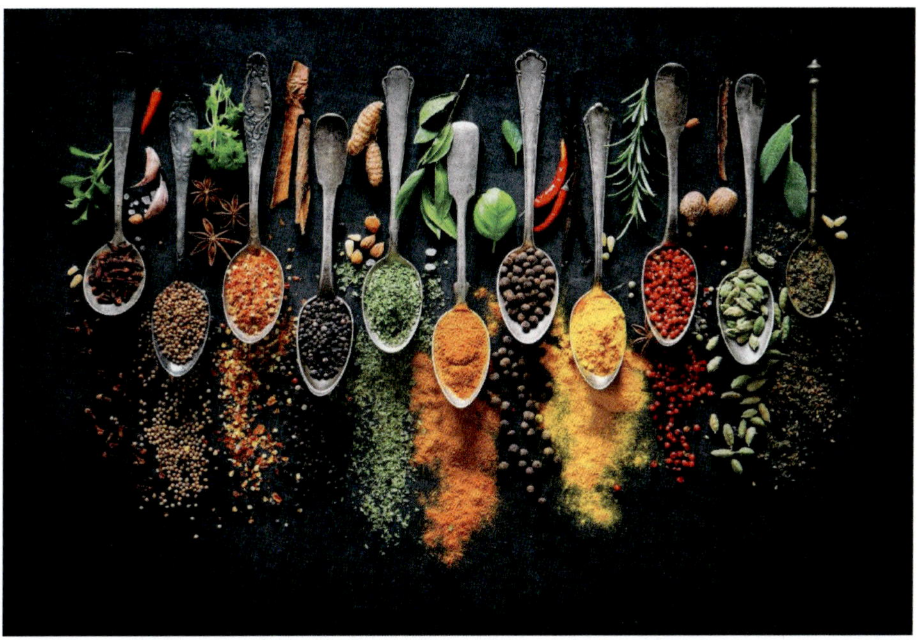

Figure 19: A selection of *phytochemical-rich* and *nutrigenomically-active* and herbs and spices

CHAPTER 14

Putting it all together

If you're now better acquainted with your cells and their pivotal role in your own health, I've achieved my primary goal in writing this book. I suggested at the outset that I would provide you with tools to help you to take back control of your health and minimise *over*-dependence on mainstream medicine.

Our journey together in exploring the emerging science of Nutrigenomics has taken us to places where few others have ventured. This is because much of the best scientific research findings remain on dusty library shelves, never to be translated into the type of simple and practical guidelines we can use in day-to-day health care. Although its focus is on Nutrigenomics, this book has gathered data from a broad base, some of which is the intermingling of my own clinical experience gained over 30 or so years in clinical practice.

From that experience, I *KNOW* that sick people can become well by embracing the principles of Nutritional Medicine; I know too that for the day-to-day ailments that fill the seats in most medical waiting rooms, the pharmaceutical drugs and surgery of mainstream medicine are best left as the *weapons of last resort*.

Unfortunately, a GP is likely to tell you that he or she is too busy to investigate a patient's diet and lifestyle in a standard five- or ten-minute consultation – and that would be right! If he were a little more honest with you (and himself), he would say he is just not trained in this area – and if he really wanted to confront the *absolute* truth, he would say that he doesn't consider much outside what his training provided. And by 'training', I refer as well to the ongoing reinforcement of these principles via the regular visits from the pharmaceutical industry's sales force.

So, how does an ordinary family get a more balanced view on practical health care, the sort of information that can help to prevent the *diseases of civilisation* to which so many of us succumb? With global budgets collapsing under the financial weight of health (or disease) expenditure, why aren't we taught how to *really* prevent illness?

To some extent, this is due to the politics of health care (*read dollars!!*). However, it is also due to the huge philosophical divide which separates the practice of mainstream medicine and the preventive strategies proposed by this book with its suggestion that better-informed individuals have more choices for their health care.

We have focused on sulforaphane and SOD as our main avenues for enhancing cellular defence because there is considerable research to support their use - and also because they can be readily incorporated into an individual's daily routine in manageable doses. Because sulforaphane can be obtained through carefully-manufactured high-yielding broccoli sprout powder or capsules, it is possible to consume it regularly. Sulforaphane exhibits broad-spectrum activity that we have only just touched on in this book. In addition to its role in 'switching on' or 'turning up' the cellular defence genes, its actions include many other protective roles.

With its safety[88] in humans confirmed, sulforaphane stands *head and shoulders* above the many popular but poorly-bioavailable supplements that marketers have exploited on the basis of *test tube* and not human clinical trials. As the science of sulforaphane continues to unfold, it is likely that we will continue to reaffirm its valuable role in human health and disease prevention.[89]

Accelerating research in this field is showing that nutrigenomic properties are emerging for other nutrients and food-derived compounds.

Sulforaphane has been shown to protect against DNA damage but the essential nutrients including folic acid, vitamin B12 and others have also been shown to protect against DNA damage.[90] Where we once thought B12 and folic acid were primarily associated with the development of normal red blood cells, we now know that they play other important roles within the cell. Decades ago, *Recommended Dietary Allowances* for these nutrients were set to ensure that we didn't become deficient in these nutrients because deficiency is known to lead to a type of anaemia affecting the red blood cells.

More recent research has shown that these recommended daily intake levels may be too low; in fact, they may be so low that they continue to allow DNA damage to occur even when the anaemia is prevented.[91]

It turns out that a particular gene, the *MTHFR* gene can be mutated and if an individual carries two copies of the mutated form, the effect of such damage is more severe than if only one copy carried the mutation. It now appears that these people require higher levels of the appropriate nutrients than if the gene were normal. Fortunately, testing for the *MTHFR* gene is becoming increasingly common. Variants of the normal gene are associated with such seemingly-unrelated disorders as cardiovascular disease and birth defects. But it is the more recent research which is showing us the importance of this same gene in protecting us against DNA damage. And to think that that every mouthful of food we consume contains compounds which engage in complex and intricate *'conversations'* with our genes, setting up elaborate signalling systems throughout the cell.

Ultimately, the extent to which we allow *health-promoting* or *disease-promoting* foods to talk to our genes is our individual choice! The more we learn about Nutrigenomics, the more we regain control over our own health – and that of the generations which follow us.

A sobering responsibility, isn't it?

REFERENCES

1. Hermsdorff HH, Zulet MA, Puchau B, Martinez JA. Fruit and vegetable consumption and proinflammatory gene expression from peripheral blood mononuclear cells in young adults: a translational study. *Nutr Metab (Lond).* 2010;7:42.
2. Starfield B. Is US health really the best in the world? *JAMA.* 2000;284(4):483-485.
3. Anderson JG, Abrahamson K. Your Health Care May Kill You: Medical Errors. *Stud Health Technol Inform.* 2017;234:13-17.
4. Ruff JS, Suchy AK, Hugentobler SA, et al. Human-relevant levels of added sugar consumption increase female mortality and lower male fitness in mice. *Nature communications.* 2013;4:2245-2245.
5. Prestera T, Holtzclaw WD, Zhang Y, Talalay P. Chemical and molecular regulation of enzymes that detoxify carcinogens. *Proc Natl Acad Sci U S A.* 1993;90(7):2965-2969.
6. Fimognari C. Sulforaphane as a promising molecule for fighting cancer *Mutation Research/Reviews in Mutation Research* 2007;635:90-104.
7. Liu RH. Potential synergy of phytochemicals in cancer prevention: mechanism of action. *J Nutr.* 2004;134(12 Suppl):3479S-3485S.
8. Marietta C, McGuire AL. Currents in contemporary ethics. Direct-to-consumer genetic testing: is it the practice of medicine? *The Journal of law, medicine & ethics : a journal of the American Society of Law, Medicine & Ethics.* 2009;37(2):369-374.
9. Surh Y-J. Nrf2 as a Master Redox Switch involved in turning on the cellular signalling involved in the induction of cytoprotective genes by chemopreventive phytochemicals. *Planta Med.* 2008;74:1526-1539.
10. Baldwin AS, Jr. The NF-kappa B and I kappa B proteins: new discoveries and insights. *Annual review of immunology.* 1996;14:649-683.
11. Nam NH. Naturally occurring NF-kappaB inhibitors. *Mini Rev Med Chem.* 2006;6(8):945-951.
12. Goszcz K, Deakin SJ, Duthie GG, Stewart D, Leslie SJ, Megson IL. Antioxidants in Cardiovascular Therapy: Panacea or False Hope? 2015;2(29).
13. Kabel AMJWJoN, Health. Free Radicals and Antioxidants: Role of Enzymes and Nutrition. 2014;2(3):35-38.
14. Yang KY, Lin LC, Tseng TY, Wang SC, Tsai TH. Oral bioavailability of curcumin in rat and the herbal analysis from Curcuma longa by LC-MS/MS. *J Chromatogr B Analyt Technol Biomed Life Sci.* 2007;853(1-2):183-189.
15. Zheng W, Lee SA. Well-done meat intake, heterocyclic amine exposure, and cancer risk. *Nutr Cancer.* 2009;61(4):437-446.

16. Gorelik S, Ligumsky M, Kohen R, Kanner J. A novel function of red wine polyphenols in humans: prevention of absorption of cytotoxic lipid peroxidation products. *Faseb j.* 2008;22(1):41-46.
17. Kuriyama S. The relation between green tea consumption and cardiovascular disease as evidenced by epidemiological studies. *J Nutr.* 2008;138(8):1548S-1553S.
18. Pearson KJ, Baur JA, Lewis KN, et al. Resveratrol delays age-related deterioration and mimics transcriptional aspects of dietary restriction without extending life span. *Cell metabolism.* 2008;8(2):157-168.
19. Walle T, Hsieh F, DeLegge MH, Oatis JE, Jr., Walle UK. High absorption but very low bioavailability of oral resveratrol in humans. *Drug Metab Dispos.* 2004;32(12):1377-1382.
20. Pepe S, Marasco SF, Haas SJ, Sheeran FL, Krum H, Rosenfeldt FL. Coenzyme Q10 in cardiovascular disease. *Mitochondrion.* 2007;7 Suppl:S154-167.
21. Teichert J, Hermann R, Ruus P, Preiss R. Plasma kinetics, metabolism, and urinary excretion of alpha-lipoic acid following oral administration in healthy volunteers. *J Clin Pharmacol.* 2003;43(11):1257-1267.
22. Forman HJ, Zhang H, Rinna A. Glutathione: overview of its protective roles, measurement, and biosynthesis. *Mol Aspects Med.* 2009;30(1-2):1-12.
23. Kelly FJ. Gluthathione: in defence of the lung. *Food Chem Toxicol.* 1999;37(9-10):963-966.
24. Kondo T, Hirose M, Kageyama K. Roles of oxidative stress and redox regulation in atherosclerosis. *J Atheroscler Thromb.* 2009;16(5):532-538.
25. Soliman GZ. Blood lipid peroxidation (superoxide dismutase, malondialdehyde, glutathione) levels in Egyptian type 2 diabetic patients. *Singapore Med J.* 2008;49(2):129-136.
26. Witschi A, Reddy S, Stofer B, Lauterburg BH. The systemic availability of oral glutathione. *Eur J Clin Pharmacol.* 1992;43(6):667-669.
27. Bjelakovic G, Nikolova D, Gluud LL, Simonetti RG, Gluud C. Antioxidant supplements for prevention of mortality in healthy participants and patients with various diseases. *Sao Paulo Med J.* 2015;133(2):164-165.
28. Omenn GS, Goodman GE, Thornquist MD, et al. Risk factors for lung cancer and for intervention effects in CARET, the Beta-Carotene and Retinol Efficacy Trial. *J Natl Cancer Inst.* 1996;88(21):1550-1559.
29. Ristow M, Zarse K, Oberbach A, et al. Antioxidants prevent health-promoting effects of physical exercise in humans. *Proc Natl Acad Sci U S A.* 2009;106(21):8665-8670.
30. Zhang Q, Pi J, Woods CG, Andersen ME. A systems biology perspective on Nrf2-mediated antioxidant response. *Toxicology and Applied Pharmacology.* 2010;244(1):84-97.

31. Agarwal M, Mehta PK, Dwyer JH, et al. Differing Relations to Early Atherosclerosis between Vitamin C from Supplements vs. Food in the Los Angeles Atherosclerosis Study: A Prospective Cohort Study. *Open Cardiovasc Med J.* 2012;6:113-121.
32. Brownlee M. The pathobiology of diabetic complications: a unifying mechanism. *Diabetes.* 2005;54(6):1615-1625.
33. Baines KJ, Wood LG, Gibson PG. The nutrigenomics of asthma: molecular mechanisms of airway neutrophilia following dietary antioxidant withdrawal. *Omics : a journal of integrative biology.* 2009;13(5):355-365.
34. Zalba G, Fortuno A, San Jose G, Moreno MU, Beloqui O, Diez J. Oxidative stress, endothelial dysfunction and cerebrovascular disease. *Cerebrovasc Dis.* 2007;24 Suppl 1:24-29.
35. Hu R, Xu C, Shen G, et al. Gene expression profiles induced by cancer chemopreventive isothiocyanate sulforaphane in the liver of C57BL/6J mice and C57BL/6J/Nrf2 (-/-) mice. *Cancer Lett.* 2006;243(2):170-192.
36. Fahey JW, Kensler TW. Role of dietary supplements/nutraceuticals in chemoprevention through induction of cytoprotective enzymes. *Chem Res Toxicol.* 2007;20(4):572-576.
37. Petri N, Tannergren C, Holst B, et al. Absorption/metabolism of sulforaphane and quercetin, and regulation of phase II enzymes, in human jejunum in vivo. *Drug Metab Dispos.* 2003;31(6):805-813.
38. Chen XL, Kunsch C. Induction of cytoprotective genes through Nrf2/antioxidant response element pathway: a new therapeutic approach for the treatment of inflammatory diseases. *Curr Pharm Des.* 2004;10(8):879-891.
39. Talalay P, Fahey JW. Phytochemicals from cruciferous plants protect against cancer by modulating carcinogen metabolism. *J Nutr.* 2001;131(11 Suppl):3027S-3033S.
40. Piao CS, Gao S, Lee GH, et al. Sulforaphane protects ischemic injury of hearts through antioxidant pathway and mitochondrial K(ATP) channels. *Pharmacol Res.* 2009.
41. Brown RH, Reynolds C, Brooker A, Talalay P, Fahey JW. Sulforaphane improves the bronchoprotective response in asthmatics through Nrf2-mediated gene pathways. *Respir Res.* 2015;16:106.
42. Vauzour D, Buonfiglio M, Corona G, et al. Sulforaphane protects cortical neurons against 5-S-cysteinyl-dopamine-induced toxicity through the activation of ERK1/2, Nrf-2 and the upregulation of detoxification enzymes. 2010;54(4):532-542.
43. Yanaka A, Fahey JW, Fukumoto A, et al. Dietary sulforaphane-rich broccoli sprouts reduce colonization and attenuate gastritis in Helicobacter pylori-infected mice and humans. *Cancer Prev Res (Phila Pa).* 2009;2(4):353-360.

44. Singh K, Connors SL, Macklin EA, et al. Sulforaphane treatment of autism spectrum disorder (ASD). *Proc Natl Acad Sci U S A.* 2014;111(43):15550-15555.
45. Bahadoran Z, Mirmiran P, Hosseinpanah F, Rajab A, Asghari G, Azizi F. Broccoli sprouts powder could improve serum triglyceride and oxidized LDL/LDL-cholesterol ratio in type 2 diabetic patients: A randomized double-blind placebo-controlled clinical trial. *Diabetes Res Clin Pract.* 2012.
46. Mirmiran P, Bahadoran Z, Hosseinpanah F, Keyzad A, Azizi F. Effects of broccoli sprout with high sulforaphane concentration on inflammatory markers in type 2 diabetic patients: A randomized double-blind placebo-controlled clinical trial. *Journal of Functional Foods.* 2012;4(4):837-841.
47. Zhang Y, Talalay P, Cho CG, Posner GH. A major inducer of anticarcinogenic protective enzymes from broccoli: isolation and elucidation of structure. *Proc Natl Acad Sci U S A.* 1992;89(6):2399-2403.
48. He X, Kan H, Cai L, Ma Q. Nrf2 is critical in defense against high glucose-induced oxidative damage in cardiomyocytes. *J Mol Cell Cardiol.* 2009;46(1):47-58.
49. Rungapamestry V, Duncan AJ, Fuller Z, Ratcliffe B. Effect of meal composition and cooking duration on the fate of sulforaphane following consumption of broccoli by healthy human subjects. *Br J Nutr.* 2007;97(4):644-652.
50. Fahey JW, Zhang Y, Talalay P. Broccoli sprouts: an exceptionally rich source of inducers of enzymes that protect against chemical carcinogens. *Proc Natl Acad Sci U S A.* 1997;94(19):10367-10372.
51. Matusheski NV, Swarup R, Juvik JA, Mithen R, Bennett M, Jeffery EH. Epithiospecifier protein from broccoli (Brassica oleracea L. ssp. italica) inhibits formation of the anticancer agent sulforaphane. *J Agric Food Chem.* 2006;54(6):2069-2076.
52. West LG, Meyer KA, Balch BA, Rossi FJ, Schultz MR, Haas GW. Glucoraphanin and 4-hydroxyglucobrassicin contents in seeds of 59 cultivars of broccoli, raab, kohlrabi, radish, cauliflower, brussels sprouts, kale, and cabbage. *J Agric Food Chem.* 2004;52(4):916-926.
53. Kushad MM, Brown AF, Kurilich AC, et al. Variation of glucosinolates in vegetable crops of Brassica oleracea. *J Agric Food Chem.* 1999;47(4):1541-1548.
54. Kensler TW, Wakabayashi N, Biswal S. Cell survival responses to environmental stresses via the Keap1-Nrf2-ARE pathway. *Annu Rev Pharmacol Toxicol.* 2007;47:89-116.
55. Andriollo-Sanchez M, Hininger-Favier I, Meunier N, et al. Age-related oxidative stress and antioxidant parameters in middle-aged and older European subjects: the ZENITH study. *Eur J Clin Nutr.* 2005;59 Suppl 2:S58-62.

56. Huber W. Orgotein--(bovine Cu-Zn superoxide dismutase), an anti-inflammatory protein drug: discovery, toxicology and pharmacology. *Eur J Rheumatol Inflamm.* 1981;4(2):173-182.
57. Vouldoukis I, Lacan D, Kamate C, et al. Antioxidant and anti-inflammatory properties of a Cucumis melo LC. extract rich in superoxide dismutase activity. *J Ethnopharmacol.* 2004;94(1):67-75.
58. Vouldoukis I, Conti M, Krauss P, et al. Supplementation with gliadin-combined plant superoxide dismutase extract promotes antioxidant defences and protects against oxidative stress. *Phytother Res.* 2004;18(12):957-962.
59. Muth CM, Glenz Y, Klaus M, Radermacher P, Speit G, Leverve X. Influence of an orally effective SOD on hyperbaric oxygen-related cell damage. *Free Radic Res.* 2004;38(9):927-932.
60. Bader N, Bosy-Westphal A, Koch A, Mueller MJ. Influence of vitamin C and E supplementation on oxidative stress induced by hyperbaric oxygen in healthy men. *Annals of nutrition & metabolism.* 2006;50(3):173-176.
61. Cloarec M, Caillard P, Provost JC, Dever JM, Elbeze Y, Zamaria N. GliSODin, a vegetal sod with gliadin, as preventative agent vs. atherosclerosis, as confirmed with carotid ultrasound-B imaging. *Allerg Immunol (Paris).* 2007;39(2):45-50.
62. Lonn E. Carotid artery intima-media thickness--a new noninvasive gold standard for assessing the anatomic extent of atherosclerosis and cardiovascular risk? *Clin Invest Med.* 1999;22(4):158-160.
63. Crouse JR, 3rd, Raichlen JS, Riley WA, et al. Effect of rosuvastatin on progression of carotid intima-media thickness in low-risk individuals with subclinical atherosclerosis: the METEOR Trial. *JAMA.* 2007;297(12):1344-1353.
64. Gutteridge JM, Halliwell B. Antioxidants: Molecules, medicines, and myths. *Biochemical and biophysical research communications.* 2010;393(4):561-564.
65. Lohwasser C, Neureiter D, Weigle B, Kirchner T, Schuppan D. The receptor for advanced glycation end products is highly expressed in the skin and upregulated by advanced glycation end products and tumor necrosis factor-alpha. *J Invest Dermatol.* 2006;126(2):291-299.
66. Mac-Mary S, Sainthillier JM, Courderotmasuyer C, Creidi P, Humbert P. Could a photobiological test be a suitable method to assess the anti-oxidant effect of a nutritional supplement Glisodin? *Eur J Dermatol.* 2007;17(3):254-255.
67. Kim HJ, Barajas B, Wang M, Nel AE. Nrf2 activation by sulforaphane restores the age-related decrease of T(H)1 immunity: role of dendritic cells. *J Allergy Clin Immunol.* 2008;121(5):1255-1261.e1257.
68. Guzik TJ, West NE, Black E, et al. Vascular superoxide production by NAD(P)H oxidase: association with endothelial dysfunction and clinical risk factors. *Circulation research.* 2000;86(9):E85-90.

69. Kern DG, Draelos ZD, Meadows C, James Morre D, Morre DM. Controlling reactive oxygen species in skin at their source to reduce skin aging. *Rejuvenation research.* 2010;13(2-3):165-167.
70. Zhang JC, Yao W, Dong C, et al. Prophylactic effects of sulforaphane on depression-like behavior and dendritic changes in mice after inflammation. *J Nutr Biochem.* 2017;39:134-144.
71. Zhang JC, Yao W, Dong C, et al. Corrigendum to "Prophylactic Effects of Sulforaphane on Depression-Like Behavior and Dendritic Changes in Mice After Inflammation" [Journal of Nutritional Biochemistry; 39(2017); 134-144]. *J Nutr Biochem.* 2021;89:108562.
72. Wu C, Chen X, Lai J, Xu Y, Hu S. The efficacy and safety of sulforaphane as an adjuvant in the treatment of bipolar depressive disorder: Study protocol for a randomized, double-blinded, placebo-controlled, parallel-group clinical trial. 2020;99(26):e20981.
73. Heber D, Li Z, Garcia-Lloret M, et al. Sulforaphane-rich broccoli sprout extract attenuates nasal allergic response to diesel exhaust particles. *Food Funct.* 2014;5(1):35-41.
74. Riedl MA, Saxon A, Diaz-Sanchez D. Oral sulforaphane increases Phase II antioxidant enzymes in the human upper airway. *Clin Immunol.* 2009;130(3):244-251.
75. Yanaka A, Fahey JW, Fukumoto A, et al. Dietary sulforaphane-rich broccoli sprouts reduce colonization and attenuate gastritis in Helicobacter pylori-infected mice and humans. *Cancer Prev Res (Phila).* 2009;2(4):353-360.
76. Egner PA, Chen JG, Wang JB, et al. Bioavailability of Sulforaphane from two broccoli sprout beverages: results of a short-term, cross-over clinical trial in Qidong, China. *Cancer Prev Res (Phila).* 2011;4(3):384-395.
77. Bahadoran Z, Mirmiran P, Hosseinpanah F, Rajab A, Asghari G, Azizi F. Broccoli sprouts powder could improve serum triglyceride and oxidized LDL/LDL-cholesterol ratio in type 2 diabetic patients: a randomized double-blind placebo-controlled clinical trial. *Diabetes Res Clin Pract.* 2012;96(3):348-354.
78. Bahadoran Z, Tohidi M, Nazeri P, Mehran M, Azizi F, Mirmiran P. Effect of broccoli sprouts on insulin resistance in type 2 diabetic patients: a randomized double-blind clinical trial. *Int J Food Sci Nutr.* 2012;63(7):767-771.
79. Cipolla BG, Mandron E, Lefort JM, et al. Effect of Sulforaphane in Men with Biochemical Recurrence after Radical Prostatectomy. *Cancer Prev Res (Phila).* 2015;8(8):712-719.
80. Galan MV, Kishan AA, Silverman AL. Oral broccoli sprouts for the treatment of Helicobacter pylori infection: a preliminary report. *Dig Dis Sci.* 2004;49(7-8):1088-1090.

81. Lopez-Chillon MT, Carazo-Diaz C, Prieto-Merino D, Zafrilla P, Moreno DA, Villano D. Effects of long-term consumption of broccoli sprouts on inflammatory markers in overweight subjects. *Clin Nutr.* 2018.
82. Yanaka A. Sulforaphane enhances protection and repair of gastric mucosa against oxidative stress in vitro, and demonstrates anti-inflammatory effects on Helicobacter pylori-infected gastric mucosae in mice and human subjects. *Curr Pharm Des.* 2011;17(16):1532-1540.
83. Murashima M, Watanabe S, Zhuo XG, Uehara M, Kurashige A. Phase 1 study of multiple biomarkers for metabolism and oxidative stress after one-week intake of broccoli sprouts. *Biofactors.* 2004;22(1-4):271-275.
84. Atwell LL, Hsu A, Wong CP, et al. Absorption and chemopreventive targets of sulforaphane in humans following consumption of broccoli sprouts or a myrosinase-treated broccoli sprout extract. *Mol Nutr Food Res.* 2015;59(3):424-433.
85. Chang YW, Jang JY, Kim YH, Kim JW, Shim JJ. The Effects of Broccoli Sprout Extract Containing Sulforaphane on Lipid Peroxidation and Helicobacter pylori Infection in the Gastric Mucosa. *Gut and liver.* 2015;9(4):486-493.
86. Ding L-A, Li J-S. Gut in diseases: physiological elements and their clinical significance. *World journal of gastroenterology.* 2003;9(11):2385-2389.
87. Suez J, Zmora N, Segal E, Elinav E. The pros, cons, and many unknowns of probiotics. *Nature Medicine.* 2019;25(5):716-729.
88. Shapiro TA, Fahey JW, Dinkova-Kostova AT, et al. Safety, tolerance, and metabolism of broccoli sprout glucosinolates and isothiocyanates: a clinical phase I study. *Nutr Cancer.* 2006;55(1):53-62.
89. Mutch DM, Wahli W, Williamson G. Nutrigenomics and nutrigenetics: the emerging faces of nutrition. *FASEB J.* 2005;19(12):1602-1616.
90. Bull C, Fenech M. Genome-health nutrigenomics and nutrigenetics: nutritional requirements or 'nutriomes' for chromosomal stability and telomere maintenance at the individual level. *Proc Nutr Soc.* 2008;67(2):146-156.
91. Fenech MF. Dietary reference values of individual micronutrients and nutriomes for genome damage prevention: current status and a road map to the future. *The American journal of clinical nutrition.* 2010;91(5):1438S-1454S.

A smaller version of this image appeared within the text on page 89

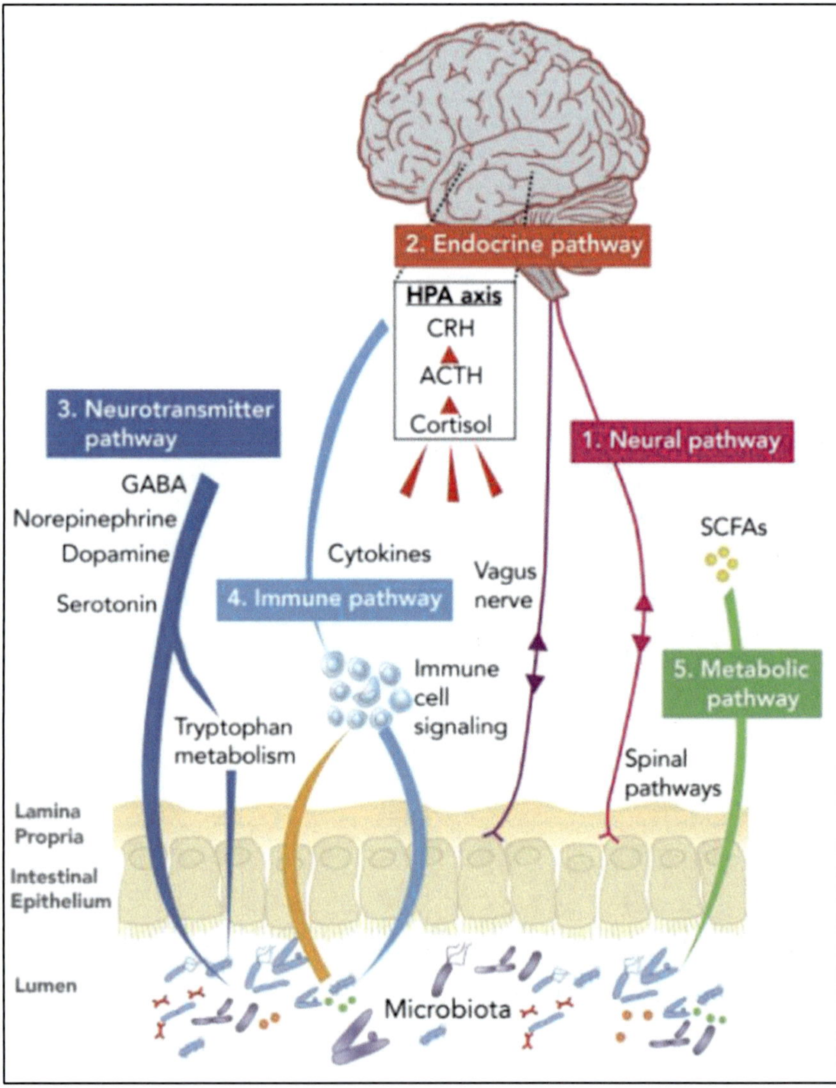

Figure 18: The Gut-Brain Axis as an example of the complex signalling that occurs between the Gut-Immune Interface and the brain.

My Notes

Made in the USA
Monee, IL
25 June 2025

20008024R00064